CALCIUM REGULATION
IN BIOLOGICAL SYSTEMS

PROCEEDINGS OF THE SECOND TAKEDA SYMPOSIUM ON BIOSCIENCE—1983

Members of the Symposium Committee

Setsuro Ebashi

*National Institute for
Physiological Sciences,
Okazaki, Japan*

Osamu Hayaishi

*Osaka Medical College
Takatsuki, Japan*

Tomoji Suzuki

*Kyoto University
Kyoto, Japan*

Hamao Umezawa

*Institute of Microbial Chemistry
Tokyo, Japan*

Yuichi Yamamura

*Osaka University
Osaka, Japan*

CALCIUM
REGULATION
IN BIOLOGICAL
SYSTEMS

Edited by

Setsuro Ebashi

National Institute for Physiological Sciences
Okazaki, Japan

Makoto Endo

The University of Tokyo
Tokyo, Japan

Kazutomo Imahori

Tokyo Metropolitan Institute of Gerontology
Tokyo, Japan

Shiro Kakiuchi

Osaka University
Osaka, Japan

Yasutomi Nishizuka

Kobe University
Kobe, Japan

1984

ACADEMIC PRESS
(Harcourt Brace Jovanovich, Publishers)

Tokyo   Orlando   San Diego   New York
London   Toronto   Montreal   Sydney

ACADEMIC PRESS RAPID MANUSCRIPT REPRODUCTION

Proceedings of the Second Takeda Science Foundation
Symposium on Bioscience, 1983
Held in Kyoto, Japan
November 21–23, 1983

ACADEMIC PRESS JAPAN, INC.
Hokoku Bldg. 3-11-13, Iidabashi, Chiyoda-ku, Tokyo 102

United States Edition published by ACADEMIC PRESS, INC.
Orlando, Florida 32887

United Kingdom Edition published by ACADEMIC PRESS, INC. (LONDON) LTD.
24/28 Oval Road, London NW1 7DX

Library of Congress Cataloging in Publication Data

Main entry under title:

Calcium regulation in biological systems.

    Proceedings of the Second Takeda Science Foundation
Symposium on Bioscience, held Nov. 21-23, 1983 in
Kyoto, Japan.
    Includes index.
    1. Calcium--Physiological effect--Congresses.
2. Calcium--Metabolism--Regulation--Congresses.
3. Ion channels--Congresses. I. Ebashi, Setsuro,
DATE   . II. Takeda Kagaku Shinko Zaidan.
III. Takeda Science Foundation Symposium on Bioscience
(2nd : 1983 : Kyoto, Japan) [DNLM: 1. Calcium--metabolism
--congresses. W3 TA163M 2nd 1983c / QV 276 C1445]

QP535.C2C266 1984   574.19'214   84-45821
ISBN 0-12-228650-2 (U.S. : alk paper)

CONTENTS

I. REGULATION OF CELLULAR FUNCTIONS BY CALCIUM IONS

II. CALCIUM CHANNEL AND TRANSMEMBRANE CONTROL

III. CALCIUM DEPENDENT PROTEASE

CONTRIBUTORS

Numbers in parentheses indicate the pages on which the authors' contributions begin.

Alastair Aitken (29), *Department of Pharmaceutical Chemistry, School of London, London WC1N 1AX, England*

Vickie E. Baracos (227), *Department of Physiology and Biophysics, Harvard Medical School, Boston, Massachusetts 02115*

Arthur M. Brown (171), *Department of Physiology and Biophysics, University of Texas Medical Branch, Galveston, Texas 77550*

Philip Cohen (29), *Department of Biochemistry, University of Dundee, Scotland*

Setsuro Ebashi (59), *National Institute for Physiological Sciences, Okazaki 444, Japan*

Makoto Endo (197), *Department of Pharmacology, Faculty of Medicine, University of Tokyo, Tokyo 113, Japan*

John H. Exton (141), *Howard Hughes Medical Institute and Department of Physiology, Vanderbilt University School of Medicine, Nashville, Tennessee 37232*

Hitoshi Fujisawa (129), *Department of Biochemistry, Asahikawa Medical College, Asahikawa 078-11, Japan*

Alfred L. Goldberg (227), *Department of Physiology and Biophysics, Harvard Medical School, Boston, Massachusetts 02115*

Robert E. Greenberg (227), *Department of Pediatrics, University of New Mexico, Albuquerque, New Mexico 87131*

Koichi Hagiwara (243), *Division of Neuromuscular Research, National Center for Nervous, Mental, and Muscular Disorders, Tokyo 187, Japan*

David J. Hartshorne (41), *Muscle Biology Group, University of Arizona, Tucson, Arizona 85721*

Philip T. Hawkins (85), *Department of Biochemistry, University of Birmingham, Birmingham B15 2TT, England*

John N. Hawthorne (117), *Department of Biochemistry, University Hospital and Medical School, Nottingham NG7 2UH, England*

Mitsuo Ikebe (41), *Department of Biochemistry, University of Dundee, Scotland*

vii

Kazutomo Imahori (213), *Department of Biochemistry, Tokyo Metropolitan Institute of Gerontology, Tokyo 173, Japan*

Shoichi Ishiura (243), *Division of Neuromuscular Research, National Center for Nervous, Mental, and Muscular Disorders, Tokyo 187, Japan*

Kozo Kaibuchi (105), *Department of Biochemistry, Kobe University School of Medicine, Kobe 650, Japan*

Keiko Kamakura (243), *Division of Neuromuscular Research, National Center for Nervous, Mental, and Muscular Disorders, Tokyo 187, Japan*

Toshiaki Katada (157), *Department of Physiological Chemistry, Faculty of Pharmaceutical Sciences, Hokkaido University, Sapporo 060, Japan*

Yuko Katakami (105), *Department of Biochemistry, Kobe University School of Medicine, Kobe 650, Japan*

Seiichi Kawashima (213), *Department of Biochemistry, Tokyo Metropolitan Institute of Gerontology, Tokyo 173, Japan*

Ushio Kikkawa (105), *Department of Biochemistry, Kobe University School of Medicine, Kobe 650, Japan*

Christopher J. Kirk (85), *Department of Biochemistry, University of Birmingham, Birmingham B15 2TT, England*

Claude B. Klee (29), *Laboratory of Biochemistry, National Cancer Institute, National Institutes of Health, Bethesda, Maryland 20205*

Robert H. Kretsinger (1), *Department of Biology, University of Virginia, Charlottesville, Virginia 22901*

Marie H. Krinks (29), *Laboratory of Biochemistry, National Cancer Institute, National Institutes of Health, Bethesda, Maryland 20205*

Allan S. Manalan (29), *Laboratory of Biochemistry, National Cancer Institute, National Institutes of Health, Bethesda, Maryland 20205*

Robert H. Michell (85), *Department of Biochemistry, University of Birmingham, Birmingham B15 2TT, England*

Osamu Minowa (17), *Department of Chemistry, Faculty of Science, Hokkaido University, Sapporo 060, Japan*

Toshihiko Murayama (157), *Department of Physiological Chemistry, Faculty of Pharmaceutical Sciences, Hokkaido University, Sapporo 060, Japan*

Tsutomu Nakamura (157), *Department of Physiological Chemistry, Faculty of Pharmaceutical Sciences, Hokkaido University, Sapporo 060, Japan*

Hirofumi Nakase (243), *Division of Neuromuscular Research, National Center for Nervous, Mental, and Muscular Disorders, Tokyo 187, Japan*

Hiroyasu Nakata (129), *Department of Biochemistry, Asahikawa Medical College, Asahikawa 078-11, Japan*

Yasutomi Nishizuka (105), *Department of Biochemistry, Kobe University School of Medicine, Kobe 650, Japan*

Ikuya Nonaka (243), *Division of Ultrastructural Research, National Center for Nervous, Mental, and Muscular Disorders, Tokyo 187, Japan*

Yoshiaki Nonomura (59), *Department of Pharmacology, Faculty of Medicine, University of Tokyo, Tokyo 113, Japan*

Harunori Ohmori (185), *Department of Neurobiology, Brain Research Institute, Faculty of Medicine, University of Tokyo, Tokyo 113, Japan*

Sachiko Okuno (129), *Department of Biochemistry, Asahikawa Medical College, Asahikawa 078-11, Japan*

Sue Palmer (85), *Department of Biochemistry, University of Birmingham, Birmingham B15 2TT, England*

Thomas D. Pollard (71), *Department of Cell Biology and Anatomy, Johns Hopkins Medical School, Baltimore, Maryland 21205*

Makoto Sawamura (105), *Department of Biochemistry, Kobe University School of Medicine, Kobe 650, Japan*

Hideo Sugita (243), *Division of Neuromuscular Research, National Center for Nervous, Mental, and Muscular Disorders, Tokyo 187, Japan*

Koichi Suzuki (213), *Department of Molecular Genetics, Tokyo Metropolitan Institute of Medical Science, Tokyo 113, Japan*

Abdel-Mohsen F. Swilem (117), *Department of Biochemistry, University Hospital and Medical School, Nottingham NG7 2UH, England*

Yoshimi Takai (105), *Department of Biochemistry, Kobe University School of Medicine, Kobe 650, Japan*

Ken-ichi Tomomatsu (243), *First Department of Internal Medicine, Faculty of Medicine, University of Tokyo, Tokyo 113, Japan*

Michio Ui (157), *Department of Physiological Chemistry, Faculty of Pharmaceutical Sciences, Hokkaido University, Sapporo 060, Japan*

Koichi Yagi (17), *Department of Chemistry, Faculty of Science, Hokkaido University, Sapporo 060, Japan*

Takashi Yamauchi (129), *Department of Biochemistry, Asahikawa Medical College, Asahikawa 078-11, Japan*

Michio Yazawa (17), *Department of Chemistry, Faculty of Science, Hokkaido University, Sapporo 060, Japan*

Mikiharu Yoshida (17), *Department of Chemistry, Faculty of Science, Hokkaido University, Sapporo 060, Japan*

FOREWORD

The Takeda Science Foundation was established in 1963 by the late Mr. Chobei Takeda VI—former President of the Takeda Chemical Industries, Ltd. and the first chairman of the foundation—through an endowment from the Takeda Chemical Industries, Ltd. The foundation was created to promote and support studies on science and technology that would contribute to the advancement of science throughout the world. During the intervening 20 years, several activities were undertaken to achieve this goal.

One of these activities, planned in 1981, was the convening of an annual Takeda Science Foundation Symposium on Bioscience under the supervision of a symposium committee organized by Setsuro Ebashi, M.D. (Professor, University of Tokyo, now Professor Emeritus; Professor, National Institute for Physiological Sciences, Okazaki); Osamu Hayaishi, M.D. (Professor, Kyoto University, now Professor Emeritus; President, Osaka Medical College); Tomoji Suzuki, Ph.D. (Professor Emeritus, Kyoto University); Hamao Umezawa, M.D. (Professor Emeritus, University of Tokyo; Director, Institute of Microbial Chemistry); and Yuichi Yamamura, M.D. (President, Osaka University).

The foundation hoped that these symposia would contribute to the promotion of international cooperation in solving many problems in the biosciences. The first symposium was held successfully in 1982. We were pleased to hold the Second Takeda Science Foundation Symposium on Bioscience 1983, entitled "Calcium Regulation in Biological Systems," on November 21–23, 1983, in Kyoto. The proceedings constitute this volume, which was edited for publication by the Organizing Committee chaired by Dr. S. Ebashi.

We are very grateful to the members of the Symposium Committee for supervising the Second Symposium, and we express our hearty thanks to the members of the Organizing Committee for planning such an excellent program and making the symposium successful.

SUEO TATSUOKA, PH.D.
Chairman, the Board of Trustees
Takeda Science Foundation

PREFACE

The motivation for this book was an international symposium held in Kyoto, Japan in November 1983, on regulatory mechanisms mediated by calcium ions. The view that the calcium ion is the most important fundamental regulating factor for various intracellular processes of all cells is acquiring citizenship in the biological sciences.

We can find several precedents for an investigation, first conducted on skeletal muscle, which has opened a new front in biology. This is also true of the regulatory role of calcium ion. The first suggestion along this line was made intuitively by L. V. Heilbrunn around 1940 using frog skeletal muscle. This inspired T. Kamada who, in collaboration with H. Kinosita (1943), carried out the experiment detecting localized, reversible contracture by injecting Ca into the cytoplasm of a muscle fiber through a micropipette. Strangely, this work even with a similar experiment by Heilbrunn and F. J. Wiercinski in 1947, did not arouse the interest of muscle scientists in calcium ion, perhaps because it was surpassed by the dramatic success of the actomyosin-ATP system discovered by A. Szent-Györgyi. Fifteen years passed before the final establishment of the role of the calcium ion in muscle, as R. H. Kretsinger points out in the first chapter of this book.

Even then, the calcium ion was confined to muscle for another ten years. Its emancipation was largely due to the 1970 discovery by S. Kakiuchi and W. Y. Cheung of the miracle calcium binding protein, calmodulin, to which a large part of this book is dedicated.

As a result, the calcium ion has become the common property of biological scientists. We know now that muscle contraction is only one of numerous functions under calcium ion control.

This book should greatly enhance the level of calcium research with its presentation of the most recent findings in this area. However, this is only the beginning of the calcium era and no one yet can predict how deeply the calcium ion is actually involved in our life. It is perhaps not too bold to say that one of the most important aspects of evolution may be the attempt of living organisms to utilize the calcium ion in an increasingly sophisticated way.

The Takeda Science Foundation Symposium on Bioscience, 1983, entitled "Calcium Regulation in Biological Systems," was held November 21–23 and provided a good forum for discussion among 212 scientists from the United States, the United Kingdom, West Germany, and Japan. On behalf of the Organizing Committee, I would like to express my sincere thanks to all contributors to this volume, and to the Takeda Science Foundation for its sponsorship of the timely and valuable symposium which has led to publication of this record.

SETSURO EBASHI

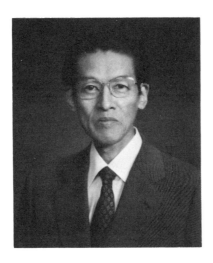

IN MEMORY OF
SHIRO KAKIUCHI
January 11, 1929–September 23, 1984

Dr. Shiro Kakiuchi, Professor of Pharmacology and Biochemistry, Institute of Higher Nervous Activity, Osaka University, died of pancreatic cancer on September 23. His untimely death brought deep grief and sadness to his friends, especially the editors of this book, who collaborated with him in planning and organizing the symposium from which this book emerged. It was experienced as a great loss within the scientific community both in Japan and around the world.

Dr. Kakiuchi was born in Kanazawa City, a beautiful old city facing the Japan Sea. After receiving his M.D. from the Faculty of Medicine, Osaka University, he took the graduate course in biochemistry under the direction of Professor Katashi Ichihara, studying the metabolism of histidine. His original intention was to become a psychiatrist so he began clinical training, but his ardor for inquiring into the heart of matters compelled him to continue research work.

After receiving his doctorate, he went to the laboratory of Professor E. H. Sutherland in 1961 and worked on the cyclic AMP level in the cell. This was a milestone in his scientific career. Here he learned that an important biochemical subject would be a molecular approach to cellular regulation.

Upon his return to Japan in 1966, he was asked by Professor Isamu Sano, a psychiatrist deeply concerned with the biochemical approach to the human mind, to organize a research laboratory in Nakamiya Hospital, Osaka. What he found there was simply the space without equipment. However, since he continued to work as a physician, he could not spend his time exclusively either seeing patients or equipping the laboratory. Despite such unfavorable circumstances, he started work on brain phosphodiesterase. He continued the work here until he moved to the present position in 1976.

Although his scientific approach was confined to enzymology, he was interested and knowledgeable in other fields. He was impressed by current Japanese studies on muscle, especially Ca regulation of the contractile system, including the discovery of troponin. His interest in the Ca ion was strengthened by a paper indicating the role of the Ca ion in the activation of muscle phosphorylase b kinase (1967). He reported in Japanese that a fairly stable fraction of the brain extract later termed "modulator protein" activated phosphodiesterase (1969). Furthermore, the Ca ion seemed to be required for the enzyme activity.

Early in 1970, he visited my office and asked solemnly, "Can you believe such a crazy idea, that the Ca ion plays a physiological role in tissues other than muscle?" Soon after that, he sent his papers in English to a journal. These papers eventually appeared (1970) in the Proceedings of the Japan Academy.

Almost at the same time, Dr. W. Y. Cheung discovered the activating factor of phosphodiesterase through an entirely different approach. In a few years, this protein was linked to the Ca ion and named calmodulin. There was no doubt calmodulin and modulator protein were identical.

These events brought about a revolution in biological science. A quarter century ago, the Ca ion was notorious among biochemists; and even the muscle field, scientists were reluctant to accept the Ca concept. Today, Ca regulation is discussed as if it were an *a priori* concept of biology.

Dr. Kakiuchi underwent surgery on the very day his lecture at the symposium was scheduled (because of this and to our deep regret, we could not include his paper in this book). Although it appeared hopeless, he survived nearly a year because of his strong, fighting spirit. On August 30, 1984, he escaped from his hospital bed to chair a symposium in Tokyo of the Third International Congress of Cell Biology. As the organizer of the symposium and one of the hosts of the Congress, he felt a strong obligation to be there. Perhaps he also thought he should say good-bye to his old friends. He succumbed to the disease three weeks later after coming back to Osaka. He fought until the last moment, and on the whole, was a victor in his life.

SETSURO EBASHI

PART I.

REGULATION OF CELLULAR FUNCTIONS BY CALCIUM IONS

STRUCTURAL STUDIES OF CALCIUM-MODULATED PROTEINS PAST AND FUTURE

Robert H. Kretsinger

Department of Biology
University of Virginia
Charlottesville, Virginia

I. PERSPECTIVE

A. Calcium as a Second Messenger and Calcium Modulated Proteins

Calcium is today a most topical area of research; yet its origins go back a century to Ringer's studies of heart contractility. In 1881 he (1) described the optimal concentration of Na^+, of K^+, and of NH_4^+ ions to maintain frog heart contractility. The next year (2) he observed that "After the publication (just mentioned) I discovered that the saline solution which I had used had not been prepared with distilled water, but with pipe water supplied by the New River Water Company." Gratis they had furnished 38 mg calcium per litre of water. "I conclude, therefore, that a lime salt is necessary for the maintenance of muscular contractility of both the eel heart and frog skeleted muscle."

Locke (3) in 1894 found that he could cause the dissected frog sartorius muscle to contract by both direct electrical stimulation and via stimulation of the attached motor nerve. This latter indirect response depended critically on the presence of calcium in the bathing medium.

Only today are the mechanisms underlying Ringer's and Locke's observations becoming understood. Even so, they had the good fortune and the keen perception to find systems in which contraction and secretion could be controlled by altering the extracellular concentrations of calcium. We now know that these cytosol processes are regulated or modulated by the concentration of free Ca^{2+} ion within the cytosol. In

3

Copyright © 1984 by The Takeda Science Foundation
All rights of reproduction in any form reserved.
ISBN 0-12-228650-2

1920 Heilbrunn (4) wrote "In my work on artificial partheno-
genesis, I showed that all substances which incite the sea-
urchin egg to divide mitotically produce a marked increase in
the viscosity of the cytoplasm." Mazia, a student of
Heilbrunn, in 1937 (5) published "The Release of Calcium in
Arbacia Eggs on Fertilization". In Heilbrunn's Outline of
General Physiology (6) he stated "There is a large amount of
corroborative evidence to show that when cells are stimulated,
calcium is set free."

Douglas was interested in exocytosis. In 1961 he and
Rubin (7) wrote "Our experiments show that the excitant action
of Ach on the adrenal medulla is dependent on the presence of
calcium, and suggest that Ach evokes adrenal medullary secretion by causing calcium ions to penetrate the adrenal
medullary cortex." He later wrote "Calcium acts as a crucial
link in the process of stimulation-secretion coupling." Many
of his ideas had been inspired by work on muscle.

In 1939, Engelhardt and Ljubimowa (8) in Moscow described
an ATPase function for myosin "Thus the mineralization of
adenosinetriphosphate, often regarded as the primary exo-
thermic reaction in muscle contraction, proceeds under the
influence and with the direct participation of the proteins
considered to form the main basis of the contractile mechanism
of the muscle fiber." Bailey in 1942 (9) found that the
ATPase activity of myosin is activated by calcium. "We
suggest that the essential feature of excitation and contraction -- we cannot at present dissociate the two phases -- is
the liberation of the Ca ion in the neighborhood of the ATPase
grouping, which can thus by the almost instantaneous catalysis
of ATP breakdown make available a large amount of energy."

Ebashi still working at the Rockefeller 1961 (10) before
returning to Tokyo had "demonstrated that a purified preparation of the relaxing factor of skeletal muscle, shown by
electron microscopy to be a vesicular fraction, probably the
endoplasmic reticulum, is able to strongly bind calcium and
furthermore that this binding of calcium by the fraction
depends on the presence of ATP. We have supposed that the
calcium binding represents the physiological action, or the
mechanism of the relaxing factor. The results demonstrated in
the present paper support this concept, and suggest that the
calcium ion is the main controlling factor in muscle
contraction." Ebashi, by 1963 in Tokyo, described a "Third
Component Participating in the Superprecipitation of 'Natural
Actomyosin'." Finally, in 1967, Ebashi et al. (11) characterized "Troponin as the Ca^{++}-receptive Protein in the
Contractile System." "It is conceivable that binding and
detaching of Ca^{2+} to and from troponin might be of primary
importance in regulation of muscle contraction, i.e., some
conformational change of the troponin molecule induced by the

removal of Ca^{2+} might inhibit interaction of adjoining actin molecules with myosin and this inhibition might be cancelled by Ca^{2+}." Heilbrunn's ill-defined gel had been replaced by a specific calcium modulated protein. Finally, Ringer's observations had received a molecular interpretation.

In 1958 Rall and Sutherland (12) identified cAMP as the heat stable factor synthesized in particulate fractions of liver and muscle following additions of ATP and stimulation by epinephrine. By 1965 Sutherland and his colleagues (13) had extended his studies of cAMP to other hormone sensitive systems. "In brief summary, the hormone (the first messenger) interacts with a component of the cell membrane to initiate increased accumulation of a mediator (the second messenger), which then acts upon components of the effector cell." They anticipated the extension of this concept. "To date cyclic 3',5'-AMP is the only second messenger which has been identified. It is proposed other such messengers may exist, for example, to mediate the action of insulin, and that these may, or may not be other cyclic 3',5'-nucleotides."

In 1970 Rasmussen (14) published "Cell Communication, Calcium Ion, and Cyclic Adenosine Monophosphate" one of the most frequently cited papers in the literature of biology. He summarized his extensive review and analysis. "The basic elements of this system are two interrelated intracellular messengers, 3',5'-AMP and Ca^{2+}. Activation or excitation of the cell leads to an increase in both."

While biochemical studies on troponin progressed, Kretsinger and his colleagues determined the crystal structure of parvalbumin, now known to be a calcium modulated protein, found in the cytosol of vertebrate white muscle. In 1972 he (15) published "Gene Triplication Deduced from the Tertiary Structure of a Muscle Calcium Binding Protein" and suggested, "Both troponin and MCBP are acidic, pI about 4.5; both have high phenylalanine contents and high calcium affinities. The molecular weight of TN-C, however, is 19,000 while that of MCBP is 11,500. I consider it possible that MCBP exists in mammals in some reduplicated forms, considering its tendency to duplication." The next year Collins et al. (16) reported "The Amino Acid Sequence of Rabbit Skeletal Muscle Troponin C: Gene Duplication and Homology with Calcium-Binding Proteins from Carp and Hake Muscle." "The correspondence of α-helices and hydrophobic residues suggests that each of the four regions of TN-C has a three-dimensional structure very similar to the CD and EF regions of MCBP."

The discovery of what we now call calmodulin resulted from studies of the cyclic nucleotide phosphodiesterase system by Cheung and by Kakiuchi.

In 1967 Cheung (17) reported "Firstly a non-dialyzable substance has been obtained from the brain extract which shows no phosphodiesterase activity but is capable of activating the 'purified' enzyme. Secondly, the activity of a mixture of the crude and 'purified' enzyme is greater than the sum of the two enzymes assayed separately." He pursued the idea that the substance was a protease, since he found that rattlesnake venom could also increase phosphodiesterase activity. In early 1970 Kakiuchi and Yamazaki (18) described the metal ion requirements of brain cyclic nucleotide phosphodiesterase "... it would be highly probable that the calcium ion is controlling the phosphodiesterase activity under physiological status and thus affecting 3',5'-AMP level in the tissues in vivo." Cheung (19) then reported "... the activating agent (or activator) was probably associated with the crude enzyme. Second, this activating agent was as effective as the" (rattlesnake) "venom in stimulating the purified enzyme." "... it is conceivable that the activator may be important in regulating phosphodiesterase in vivo." Kakiuchi et al. (20) also "... found that a heat stable and nondialyzable factor, present in crude brain homogenate, ..." and added "It is uncertain, at present time, whether that PAF" (phosphodiesterase activating factor) "works on the enzyme which requires calcium ion for the activity, or that PAF plus calcium ion act upon the enzyme for the activation."

The publication during the past decade of over a thousand papers on calmodulin pays tribute to these investigators.

B. Four Domain Model of Calmodulin

Our best model of the structure of calmodulin is still that of Kretsinger and Barry (21) as initially described for troponin C, which is a homolog of and certainly near isostructural with calmodulin (Fig. 1). As initially seen in the crystal structure of parvalbumin and again more recently in intestinal calcium binding protein (22), each homolog domain consists of about thirty amino acids--ten in an α-helix, ten in a calcium binding loop, and ten in a second α-helix. Two domains of a single protein are approximately related by a two fold axis and are packed together to form a hydrophobic core. Both calmodulin and troponin-C contain four domains. Hence, the model for calmodulin consists of two pairs of domains; I, II and III, IV. This pairing, as opposed to I, III or to I, IV, is consistent with the fact that I and III and that II and IV are nearer one another in amino acid sequence. Further, we infer that a precursor, having two domains related by a two fold axis, underwent gene duplication to form calmodulin. In our model (Fig. 1) the local two fold axis of I, II is coincident with and antiparallel to that of III, IV, thereby generating approximate point group symmetry, 222. The

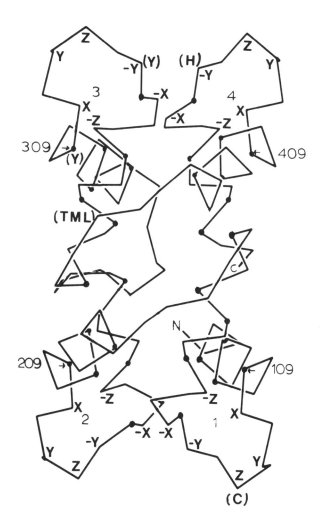

FIGURE 1. The postulated model for calmodulin consists of four homolog domains as observed in parvalbumin and in intestinal calcium binding proteins. The ninth residues of domains 1, 2, 3, and 4 are indicated. The calcium ions are coordinated by oxygen atoms of the side chains of residues 10(X), 12(Y), 14(Z), 19(-X) and 21(-Z) -- and by the peptide oxygen of 16(-Y). The residues -- 2, 5, 6, 9 and 22, 25, 26, 29 -- are hydrophobic as is the Ilu or Val at 17. These residues account for the strong affinity between domains 1 and 2 and between 3 and 4. Residues Cys (114) (of plant calmodulin), Tyr (316), trimethyllysine (325), and His (416) are indicated.

hydrophobic back sides of I, II and of III, IV, away from the Ca^{2+} ion binding loops, pack together to form an hour glass shaped molecule with a narrowed hydrophobic waist. This waist is inferred to be the site of binding to target proteins and to hydrophobic molecules such as phenothiazine.

Numerous spectroscopic experiments and chemical modification experiments are consistent with the model's having pairs of domains. Yet none of these experiments really test the most speculative part of the model, the relationship of the I, II and the III, IV domains.

C. Outstanding Questions

Numerous studies, as reviewed by Cox et al. (23) and by Seamon and Kretsinger (24), have shown that calmodulin binds four equivalents of Ca^{2+} ions with pK_d 6 to 7 under cytosolic conditions of 3.0 mM magnesium. Most of the calmodulin binding proteins, with the notable exception of phosphorylase b kinase, do not bind apo- or magnesium-calmodulin but only Ca_3^- or Ca_4^--calmodulin. It is, therefore, extremely important to understand the change(s) in conformation that accompany the binding of Ca^{2+} ions. There is, unfortunately, disagreement as to the exact values of the calcium and the magnesium binding constants. Most of these groups, as well as Delville et al. (25) who have completed extensive calculations for various models, agree that there is not a well defined sequence of site occupancy by calcium, nor that there is a significant amount of cooperativity in calcium binding.

In marked contrast, numerous spectroscopists have interpreted their studies of calcium, cadmium, or lanthanide binding to calmodulin (reviewed in References 22 and 23) in terms of a characteristic spectrum for Ca_0^-, Ca_1^-, Ca_2^-, Ca_3^-, and Ca_4^--calmodulin. Yet, at the concentration of free Ca^{2+} ion yielding maximal concentrations of Ca_2^--calmodulin, there would also be present significant amounts of Ca_1^--calmodulin and of Ca_3^--calmodulin. Further the Ca_2^--calmodulin would be present in six distinct forms with Ca^{2+} ions at sites 1 & 2, 1 & 3, 1 & 4, 2 & 3, 2 & 4, and 3 & 4. It is improbable that all six of these distinct forms, if in fact they are all present, would have the same conformation and the same spectrum.

II. STRUCTURAL STUDIES

A. Overview

Most sciences -- astronomy, geology, archeology, or biochemistry -- have a descriptive aspect. Before one can understand causal, functional, or evolutionary relationships one must identify the components of the system and their geometric relationships. In this spirit we are investigating the crystal structures of calmodulin, as well as S-100b, and the crayfish sarcoplasm calcium binding protein. We are confident that knowing these structures will not only help answer several of the outstanding questions already mentioned but also suggest new paths to follow.

B. Use of the Multiwire Area X-ray Diffractometer

Five years ago, inspired by the initial success of Xuong and coworkers (26) we decided to build a multiwire area x-ray diffractometer to function as a "Biotechnology Resource". It would, of course, facilitate our research as well as being available to all macromolecular crystallographers in America. Not surprisingly we encountered some technical problems both in hardware and in software development; however, the system is now functioning with up to four detectors measuring and integrating intensities in real time.

When a protein crystal is placed in a collimated beam of (near) monochromatic x-rays some of the sets of planes, or reciprocal lattice points, satisfy the Bragg condition and a few hundred reflections occur. As the crystal is incrementally rotated, new lattice points intersect the sphere of reflection. During a rotation of $180°/n$ (where n comes from crystal class symmetry) all, excepting a few reciprocal lattice points near the rotation axis, possible reflections will have occurred. Given such a "data set" for the native calmodulin and for several heavy atom derivatives, one can determine the crystal structure to the limit of resolution of data measured. Traditionally, crystallographers have measured these reflections one at a time on single counter diffractometers, for proteins a very slow and tedious process even on automatic diffractometers.

Each of our four detectors has an active surface area of 256 by 256 mm. Each incoming x-ray photon is counted and assigned to the nearest 1.0 mm wire in one direction and to the nearest 2.0 mm in the other. Each detector has (256 x 128 =) 32,768 memory locations in which counts from each "pixel" are accumulated. The dead time of the detector is 10^{-6} seconds. We can count up to 10^5 x-rays per second, per

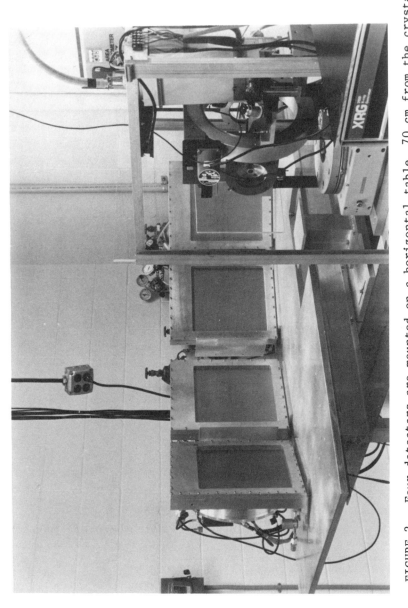

FIGURE 2. Four detectors are mounted on a horizontal table, 70 cm from the crystal. The PHI axis of the three circle goniometer is vertical. The x-ray generator is in the lower, right corner of the photograph.

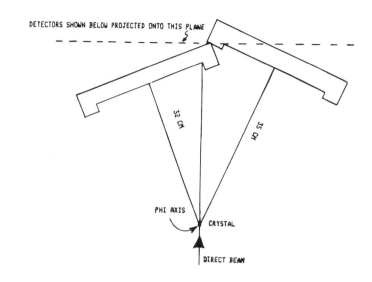

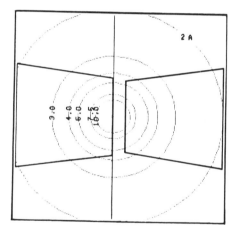

FIGURE 3. Two multiwire area x-ray detectors can measure 65% of the diffraction data from triclinic calmodulin in one total rotation of 180° (+20°) about the PHI axis of the diffractometer. In the upper figure one sees two detectors mounted on the horizontal table; their active face planes are vertical, the left at 32.0 cm, the right at 35.0 cm from the crystal. Its diffraction pattern is measured for one minute for each successive 0.08° rotation about PHI. The lower figure shows the portion of reciprocal space intercepted by the two detectors, as projected onto a plane perpendicular to the direct x-ray beam.

detector with less than 10% rejection due to coincidence. Most protein crystals, even with a rotating anode x-ray source, diffract more weakly than this.

Figure 2 shows four detectors mounted on a horizontal table. The crystal is rotated about the (near) vertical PHI axis of the three circle goniometer seen on the right side of the photograph. The detector(s) are placed on the table as close as possible to the crystal to intercept the largest possible solid angle, consistent with the constraint that individual reflections are resolved from one another.

Figure 3 shows the experimental arrangement for measuring data from crystals of calmodulin. Two detectors are placed on the table, one on either side of the direct x-ray beam, at 32.0 cm and at 35.0 cm crystal to detector distance. This arrangement permits one to measure Bijvoet pairs of reflections, or anomalous dispersion data. In order to measure all available diffraction data, we must rotate the crystal, stepwise through 180° (+20°). The step interval must be fine enough, 0.08°, to permit at least six individual measurements across a single reflection. For each of the 200° x (0.08° step^{-1})$^{-1}$ = 2,500 steps, or measurements, x-rays are counted, then assigned to background or to a particular hkl index reflection. The position of each hkl reflection is predicted in advance; a compensation is made for any small movement of the crystal. The integrated, background corrected intensities for a few degrees of rotation are calculated in real time while subsequent reflections are being measured. It requires about 1.0 minute to record highly significant data for one step, or 2,500 steps x (60 steps hr^{-1})$^{-1}$ = 42 hours to record a (near) complete set of data to nominal 2.0 Å resolution. If desired, a second 15 to 20 hour experiment with a second crystal mounted about a second crystal axis will provide the data, near the first rotation axis, which was not measured in the first experiment. There are 20,000 reciprocal lattice points (reflections) available to 2.0 Å resolution. To have measured these, one at a time with a conventional, single counter diffractometer, would have required 30,000 minutes or 500 hours.

Legend to Table I.

Crystals are grown at 4°C in a drop hanging from a coverslip over a reservoir. The contact between the coverslip and edge of the reservoir is sealed with oil so that the vapor pressures of both liquids equilibrate. The starting volume of the drop is usually near 0.020 ml and that of the reservoir 1.0 ml.

Table I. Conditions for Growth of Crystals of Calcium Modulated Proteins

Protein	Drop Conditions	Reservoir Conditions	Crystal Morphology	Space Group	Unit Cell	
Calmodulin	8% PEG 6,000 10 mM Cacodylate buffer pH 5.3 5-20 mM CaCl$_2$	25% PEG 6,000 20 mM Cacodylate buffer pH 5.3 0.5 mM β-ME	Isodimensional Irregular	P2$_1$	a b c	61.8 Å 56.7 Å 40.0 Å 92.7°
Calmodulin	6.7% PEG 6,000 6.7% MPD 20 mM Cacodylate buffer pH 5.7 20 mM CaCl$_2$	20% PEG 6,000 16.7% MPD 20 mM Cacodylate buffer pH 5.7 0.5 mM β-ME	Rods, elongated along c	P1	a b c	29.6 Å 53.8 Å 25.1 Å 93.1° 97.4° 89.9°
S-100b	10% PEG 6,000 10 mM Pipes buffer pH 5.0 0.1 mM CaCl$_2$	25% PEG 6,000 20 mM Pipes buffer pH 6.0 0.5 mM β-ME	Rods, elongated along c	P4$_1$	a b c	56.0 Å 56.0 Å 112.8 Å
CSCBP	22% MPD 10 mM Pipes buffer pH 6.5	55% MPD 20 mM Pipes buffer pH 6.5		P2$_1$2$_1$2$_1$	a b c	58.9 Å 68.5 Å 116.1 Å

C. Results of Crystallographic Studies

The great disadvantage of crystallography is the need for crystals. We spent several years defining the crystallization conditions of Table I. Perseverance and extremely pure protein proved to be the keys to success. Our first crystals of calmodulin were grown from polyethylene glycol (PEG, see table caption for details) in space group $P2_1$. As we varied the ratio of 2,4-methylpentanediol (MPD) to PEG different crystal forms with varying morphologies appeared. We have adopted as our "standard" growth conditions those of Table I. We have found that usually our calmodulin crystals are more stable in the presence of 10% more concentrated PEG/MPD than in the original growth conditions. The crystals grow larger at 4° C than at 20° C. We can however, react the crystals with heavy atoms and make the x-ray diffraction measurement at 20° C, if we first transfer the crystals to Δ10% PEG/MPD.

Obtaining usable heavy atom derivatives has proven to be especially difficult. In general, if we get occupancies approaching 1:1 stoichiometry, the crystals shatter, dissolve, and/or become very sensitive to x-radiation damage. Conversely, at the lower occupancies required for crystal stability the contribution of the heavy atom to the diffraction pattern has been so weak that we could not locate it and refine its position in difference Patterson maps.

Our experience with lanthanides has been particularly disappointing. In parvalbumin, which we crystallized from 2.8 M ammonium sulfate, the two calcium ions are readily replaced, in the crystals, by various lanthanides. When we soak calmodulin crystals in gadolinium, terbium, or praseodymium at 2.5 mM they fracture. At 1.0 mM the diffraction patterns show only very weak changes. In contrast, Szebenyi et al. (22) replaced the Ca^{2+} ion of the second domain of intestinal calcium binding protein with a Nd^{3+} ion. Both Ca^{2+} ions of crystalline parvalbumin can be replaced by Tb^{3+} ions (27). Intestinal calcium binding protein crystallizes from 3.2 M ammonium sulfate and parvalbumin from 2.8 M $(NH_4)_2SO_4$. The fracturing of crystals of calmodulin by lanthanides may reflect their having been grown in MPD/PEG or it may reflect a lack of isomorphism between calcium–calmodulin and lanthanide–calmodulin. We do not understand the implications for numerous spectroscopic studies in which lanthanides replace calcium. Horrocks and Mulqueen (MS. in preparation) have told us that in their studies of europium and calmodulin fluorescence they had to add 0.3 M NaCl to protect calmodulin from aggregation. If we increase the PEG/MPD by 40% the crystals of calmodulin can withstand 0.3 M NaCl. Unfortunately the addition of 2.5 mM lanthanides still degrades the crystals.

During the past year, while we have been completing work on the detectors and associated software, we have also completed our evaluation of promising heavy atom derivates. Over forty-five heavy atom compounds have been tested to determine their suitability as heavy atom derivatives. Most either ruined the crystals or did not react at all. However, seven -- CH_3HgCl, $Hg(CH_3CO_2^-)_2$, thimerosal, 2-hydroxymercuric-benzoate, K_2PtCl_4, H_2PtCl_6, and $Pb(CH_3CO_2^-)_2$ -- have produced significant changes in diffraction intensity. We are measuring data from these crystals using the experimental arrangement of Fig. 3.

In order to extend our evolutionary studies of the calcium modulated proteins we plan to determine the crystal structures of S-100b and of crayfish sarcoplasm calcium binding protein. Good crystals are in queue for detector time.

Compte et al. (28) have shown that calmodulin binds to melittin with K_d 10^{-9} M, the highest affinity of any calmodulin complex yet reported. We have grown small crystals of the 1:1 complex and are seeking better conditions. The next goal is an understanding of the interaction of calmodulin and its various targets.

REFERENCES

1. Ringer, S., J. Physiol. 3:195 (1881).
2. Ringer, S., J. Physiol. 4:29 (1882).
3. Locke, F. S., Zbl. Physiol. 8:166 (1894).
4. Heilbrunn, L. V., J. Exp. Zool. 30:211 (1920).
5. Mazia, D., J. Cell Comp. Physiol. 10:291 (1937).
6. Heilbrunn, L. V., "An Outline of General Physiology 3rd Edition" W. B. Saunders Co., Philadelphia, 1952.
7. Douglas, W. W., and Rubin, R. P., J. Physiol. 159:40 (1961).
8. Engelhardt, W. N., and Ljubimowa, M. N., Nature 144:668 (1939).
9. Bailey, K., Biochem. J. 36:121 (1942).
10. Ebashi, S., J. Biochem. 50:236 (1961).
11. Ebashi, S., Ebashi, F., and Kodama, A., J. Biochem. 62:137 (1967).
12. Rall, T. W., and Sutherland, E. W., J. Biol. Chem. 232:1065 (1958).
13. Sutherland, E. W., Oye, I., and Butcher, R. W., Rec. Prog. Hormone Res. 21:623 (1965).
14. Rasmussen, H., Science 170:404 (1970).
15. Kretsinger, R. H., Nature New Biol. 240:85 (1972).
16. Collins, J. H., Potter, J. D., Horn, M. J., Wilshire, G., and Jackman, H., FEBS Lett. 36:268 (1973).
17. Cheung, W. Y., Biochem. Biophys. Res. Commun. 29:478 (1967).

18. Kakiuchi, S., and Yamazaki, R., Proc. Japan Acad. 46:387 (1970).

19. Cheung, W. Y., Biochem. Biophys. Res. Commun. 38:533 (1970).

20. Kakiuchi, S., Yamazaki, R., and Nakajima, H., Proc. Japan Acad. 46:587 (1970).

21. Kretsinger, R. H., and Barry, C. D., Biochim. Biophys. Acta 405:40 (1975).

22. Szebenyi, D. M. E., Obendorf, S. K., and Moffat, K., Nature 294:327 (1981).

23. Cox, J. A., Comte, M., Malnoü, A., Burger, D., and Stein, E. A., in "Metal Ions in Biological Systems" (H. Siegel, ed.), vol. 17, p. 215. Marcel Dekker Inc., New York, 1983.

24. Seamon, K. B., and Kretsinger, R. H., in "Calcium in Biology" (T. G. Spiro, ed.), Vol. VI of Metal Ions in Biology, p. 1. John Wiley, New York, 1983.

25. Delville, A., Lasalo, P., and Nelson, D. J., J. Am. Chem. Soc. Submitted for publication.

26. Cork, C., Hamlin, R., Vernon, W., and Xuong, Ng. H., Acta Cryst. A31:702 (1975).

27. Sowadski, J., Cornick, G., and Kretsinger, R. H., J. Mol. Biol. 124:123 (1978).

28. Compte, M., Maulet, Y., and Cox, J. A., Biochem. J. 209:269 (1983).

THE HIGH AFFINITY SITES OF CALMODULIN FOR Ca^{2+} AND Mn^{2+}[1]

K. Yagi
M. Yazawa
M. Yoshida
O. Minowa

Department of Chemistry
Faculty of Science
Hokkaido University
Sapporo

I. INTRODUCTION

The primary structure of calmodulin was first determined by Vanaman et al. in 1976 (1). Since then, it has been determined with 9 different animals and a plant. Results indicate that the sequence from N-terminal acetylalanine to leucine at position 69 is identical among calmodulins isolated from animals (2).

Since the sources selected for study of the primary structure of animals cover from protozoa to vertebrata and mollusca, the animals may have held the identical structure through their evolution for about 6×10^8 years. This has occurred probably because this particular structure is indispensable for a certain crucial function of calmodulin. The N-terminal side which confines the structure is tentatively designated as N-domain, and the other half as C-domain. Each of the N- and C-domains includes two Ca^{2+}-binding sites, and either of the two may confine the high affinity sites. However, the binding of two Ca^{2+} is not sufficient to ensure activation of enzymes such as phosphodiesterase (3) and myosin

[1]This work was supported by Grant-in-Aids from the Muscular Dystrophy Association of America, Inc. and from the Ministry of Education, Science and Culture of Japan.

light chain kinase (4).   One or two more Ca^{2+}-binding to calmodulin is required.

We have stated that the high affinity sites are located on
the C-domain (5).   It then follows that saturation of the
Ca^{2+}-binding sites in C-domain is not sufficient and that
further Ca^{2+}-binding to N-domain is necessary for enzyme activation.   This leads us to the opinion that the particular
structure on N-domain plays a role in the activation.   In
order to develop this viewpoint further, it is necessary to
confirm whether the high affinity sites are really confined to
the C-domain.   Contrary results have already been presented by
Kilhoffer et al. (6) in which they concluded the N-domain to
be the high affinity sites; Wang et al. (7) and Wallace et al.
(8) have supported this conclusion.

In this paper, the results supporting our view are presented using wheat germ calmodulin which has Cys27 in N-domain
and using the proteolytic fragments of scallop testis calmodulin.   The functions of N-domain and C-domain are considered.

II. EXPERIMENTAL PROCEDURES FOR PROTEIN PREPARATIONS

Scallop testis calmodulin was isolated according to the
method of Yazawa et al. (9) and a phenyl-Sepharose column was
used for the final purification step.   The scallop calmodulin
was incubated with trypsin according to the method described
by Drabikowski et al. (10).   The incubation mixture was
applied to DEAE-cellulose and two fragments (F12 and F34) were
obtained.   F12 is equivalent to TR_1-C of bovine brain calmodulin whose sequence is from Ala1 to Arg75, and F34 is equivalent to TR_2-C whose sequence is from Asp78 to Lys148; F12
corresponds to N-domain and F34 C-domain.

Wheat germ calmodulin was isolated according to the method
of Yoshida et al. described elsewhere (11).   Protein concentrations were determined from the results of quantitative
amino acid analyses.   The known amount of norleucine was added
as the internal standard.

III. COMPARISON OF Ca^{2+}-BINDINGS OF CALMODULIN AND ITS
N-DOMAIN AND C-DOMAIN FRAGMENTS

The amount of calcium in calmodulin preparations was
measured with a Hitachi 180-30 atomic absorption spectrophotometer.

The binding of Ca^{2+} to the wheat germ and scallop testis
calmodulins was measured by the flow-dialysis method using

^{45}Ca with a Teflon apparatus as described elsewhere (12). The Ca^{2+}-binding curve of calmodulin is represented by Equation 1 derived by Adair (13),

$$r = \frac{K_1C + 2K_1K_2C^2 + 3K_1K_2K_3C^3 + 4K_1K_2K_3K_4C^4}{1 + K_1C + K_1K_2C^2 + K_1K_2K_3C^3 + K_1K_2K_3K_4C^4} \tag{1}$$

where K_1, K_2, K_3 and K_4 are the macroscopic binding constants and r the average amount of Ca^{2+} bound per mol of calmodulin at free Ca^{2+} concentration of C. Regression of data to Equation 1 was performed using a non-linear curve fitting program (14).

The average amounts of Ca^{2+} bound per mol of scallop testis and wheat germ calmodulins at various free molar Ca^{2+} concentrations are shown in Figs. 1A and B. The macroscopic binding constants best fitted to the data are calculated as shown in Table I. Lines in Fig. 1 are the representation of Equation 1 using the constants. The four values of these calmodulins were similar to the respective values of bovine brain and ram testis calmodulins (3,15).

The positive cooperativity between the first two Ca^{2+}- bindings, which was discovered by Crouch and Klee (3) with

Table I. Macroscopic Binding Constants of Ca^{2+} to Calmodulin and Its Proteolytic Fragments

	Wheat germ	Scallop testis	Bovine brain	Ram testis		Scallop testis F12	F34	Calc.
				M^{-1} x 10^{-6}				
K_1	0.25	0.34	0.3	0.5	Kc	–	0.054	0.20
K_2	0.27	0.36	0.86	0.53	Kd	–	1.92	0.60
K_3	0.12	0.13	0.12	0.14	Ka	0.147	–	0.13
K_4	0.02	0.06	0.045	0.02	Kb	0.066	–	0.06
K_5	0.015	0.0005	–	–				

The results of bovine brain (3) and ram testis (15) calmodu- lins were cited from respective references. Calc.: Calculated values using Ka, Kb, Kc and Kd.

bovine brain calmodulin, was also observed in the values of K_1 and K_2 of scallop and wheat calmodulins.

As shown in Fig. 2, the maximum amount of bound Ca^{2+} was 2 mol per mol of both F12 and F34 (16). The binding constants

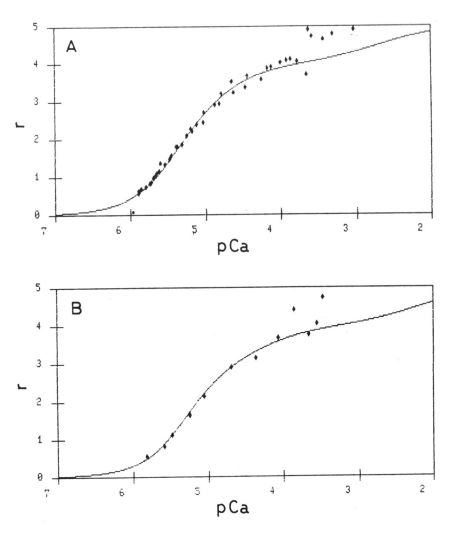

FIGURE 1. Binding of Ca^{2+} to calmodulin. Average amount of Ca^{2+} per calmodulin in molar ratio is shown against negative logarithms of free molar Ca^{2+} concentration. Solid lines are calculated from Equation 1 with the macroscopic constants given in Table I. Solvent : 0.1 M NaCl, 20 mM MOPS-NaOH (pH 7.03), at 25°C. A, Scallop testis calmodulin. B, Wheat germ calmodulin.

were calculated using Equation 2 applied for proteins with two binding sites.

$$r = \frac{K_1 c + 2K_1 K_2 c^2}{1 + K_1 c + K_1 K_2 c^2} \qquad (2)$$

The binding constants best fitted to the data are collected in Table I. Ka and Kb are the constants of F12 and Kc and Kd of F34. Lines a and b in Fig. 2 are the representation of Equation 2 using the constants. The mid points of Ca^{2+} saturation for F12 and F34 were obtained as 10.2 μM and 3.1 μM, respectively. This suggests that F12 corresponds to the half molecule containing low affinity sites and F34 high affinity sites. Since F12 is equivalent to N-domain in calmodulin, we conclude that the low affinity sites are located on N-domain and, therefore, that high affinity sites are on C-domain.

Kc and Kd were not very similar to K_1 and K_2 of a whole molecule. However, these two constants may be removed from K_1 and K_2, respectively, to the opposite direction after proteolytic separation. This tendency has been observed with troponin C (17). Since F34 shows higher affinity to Ca^{2+} than F12 and a strong positive cooperativity was demonstrated with

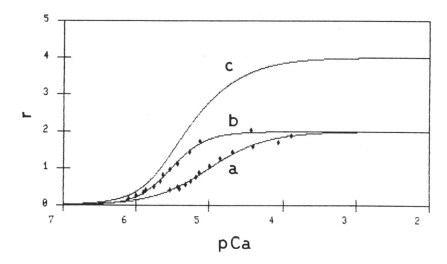

FIGURE 2. Binding of Ca^{2+} to proteolytic fragments of calmodulin. Average amount of Ca^{2+} per F12 (a) or F34 (b) in molar ratio is shown against negative logarithms of free molar Ca^{2+} concentration. Lines a and b are calculated from Equation 2 with constants given in Table I. Line c is the sum of a and b.

F34, our conclusion that Kc and Kd correspond to K_1 and K_2, respectively, may be correct.

In Fig. 2 is also shown the sum of the binding curves of F12 and F34. The macroscopic binding constants best fitted to the sum of the two curves were calculated and are summarized in Table I. The coincidence with the constants obtained from results in Fig. 1 confirms that the binding curve of calmodulin can be composed of the Ka and Kb of F12 and Kc and Kd of F34.

IV. SEPARATE DETECTION OF CONFORMATIONAL CHANGES OF N-DOMAIN AND C-DOMAIN

^{13}C-cyanylation of Cys27 of wheat calmodulin was performed with $K^{13}CN$ after the 5,5'-dithio-bis(2-nitrobenzoic acid) (DTNB) treatment (12). Lyophilized ^{13}CN-calmodulin was dissolved in 0.4 ml of D_2O containing 0.25 M KCl at pH 7.0. ^{13}C NMR spectrum was measured with a JEOL FX-100 spectrometer at 25°C. $K^{13}CN$ (99% ^{13}CN) was the product of Merck, Sharp & Dohme Canada, Ltd.

The inset in Fig. 3 shows the ^{13}C NMR spectra of ^{13}CN-calmodulin which contains 0.3 mol (a) and 3.3 mol Ca^{2+} (b) per mol. ^{13}C of the cyano group bound to Cys27 of the calmodulin gave a single peak at 114.5 ppm, and the peak position was shifted to lower magnetic field by the addition of Ca^{2+}. The changes in chemical shift were plotted against the molar ratio of added Ca^{2+} to the calmodulin (Fig. 3) (12). Practically all of the added Ca^{2+} is probably in the associated state with calmodulin under this condition. A downfield shift was found to occur with the binding of the third and fourth Ca^{2+}, indicating that the third (or fourth) Ca^{2+} binds to the site containing Cys27. Since Cys27 is involved in N-domain, the binding sites in the N-domain are the low affinity sites for Ca^{2+}.

The result of difference UV absorption spectrum induced by Ca^{2+} is also shown in Fig. 3. The difference UV absorption spectrum was recorded using a Shimadzu UV 350 recording spectrophotometer with a thermostated cell holder. The reference cell contained 0.1 mM ethyleneglycol-bis-(β-aminoethyl ether)N,N'-tetraacetic acid (EGTA) in addition to the protein solution.

The difference spectrum reflected the environmental change around Tyr139[1] which is in the C-domain. The change in dif-

---

[1]Tyr139 of wheat germ calmodulin corresponds to Tyr138 of calmodulins isolated from animals.

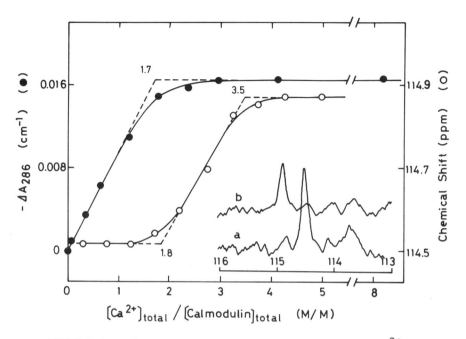

FIGURE 3. Changes in the chemical shift and Ca²⁺-induced difference UV absorption spectrum at 286 nm plotted against the molar ratio of total concentration of Ca²⁺ to ¹³CN-calmodulin. Solvent :. 0.2 M KCl, 20 mM MOPS pH 7.0, at 25°C. o, Chemical shift. •, Difference spectrum. Inset shows ¹³C NMR spectra of the calmodulin with 0.3 mol (a) and 3.3 mol (b) Ca²⁺ per mol.

ference spectrum was saturated at 1.7 mol Ca²⁺ per mol of calmodulin, suggesting that the conformational change of C-domain is accomplished by the Ca²⁺ bindings to the high affinity sites.

V. Mn²⁺-INDUCED CONFORMATIONAL CHANGES OF CALMODULIN

Spin labeling of Cys27 of wheat calmodulin was performed with N-(2,2,6,6-tetramethyl-4-piperidine-1-oxyl)maleimide purchased from Synvar, and the samples for ESR measurements were prepared as described elsewhere (11). ESR spectra were recorded at 9.21 GHz with 4 mW microwave power using a JEOL JES-FE1X with a variable temperature controller. The modulation width was 5 Gauss.

The magnitude of peak heights of ESR spectrum of spin-

labeled calmodulin decreased remarkably with the addition of
Mn^{2+}.   Line width of the peak did not change.   The quenching
may be due to the dipole–dipole interaction between the spin-
label and bound Mn^{2+}.   In Fig. 4 is shown the decrease in peak

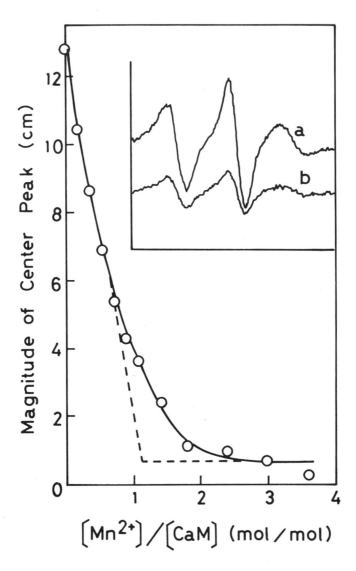

FIGURE 4.   Relation between the magnitude of center peak
and the molar ratio of added Mn^{2+} to calmodulin.   Solution
contains 83 μM calmodulin, 0.1 M NaCl, and 20 mM MOPS (pH
7.03), at 25°C.   Inset shows ESR spectra of spin-labeled
calmodulin containing 0 (a) and 75 μM (b) Mn^{2+}.

heights plotted against the added Mn^{2+} concentration (11).
The quenching of ESR spectrum became maximum with the addition
of Mn^{2+} equivalent to the calmodulin in molar ratio.   When
Ca^{2+} was added to the Mn^{2+}-calmodulin (1:1) complex, the
magnitude did not recover until the Ca^{2+} concentration reached
1.4 times that of the added Mn^{2+}.   Additional Ca^{2+} gradually
replaced Mn^{2+} which resulted in the recovery of the ESR
spectrum (11).

The difference spectrum obtained with the spin-labeled
calmodulin was identical with that of the unlabeled calmodulin. Mn^{2+} also induced a spectral shift of Tyr139 as that
Ca^{2+} induced.   The effect of added concentrations of Ca^{2+} or
Mn^{2+} on the difference absorbance measured at 286 nm was
investigated.   As shown in Fig. 5, the amount of Mn^{2+} as
necessary to attain the maximum difference absorbance was 3.2
mol per mol of calmodulin, but the amont of Ca^{2+} was 1.5 mol
per mol (11).   The excess Mn^{2+} may be attributable to the
first Mn^{2+} bound to a site different than those to Ca^{2+}.

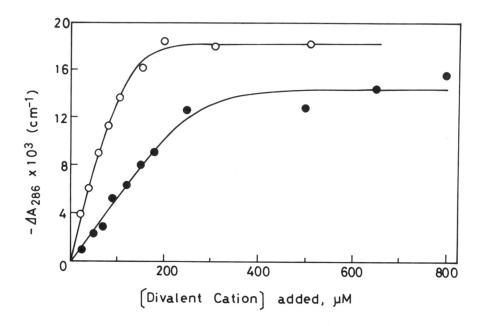

FIGURE 5.   Effect of added Ca^{2+} and Mn^{2+} concentration on
difference UV absorbance at 286 nm.   o, Ca^{2+}.   ●, Mn^{2+}.
Conditions are the same as in Fig. 4.

VI. POSSIBLE FUNCTIONS OF N-DOMAIN AND C-DOMAIN

The high affinity sites for Ca^{2+} are located on the C-domain, while Mn^{2+} first binds to the N-domain. These conclusions were deduced from the following evidence.

1) After saturation of the high affinity sites, the third Ca^{2+} binds to the site containing Cys27 (Fig. 3).
2) Mn^{2+} first binds to the site containing Cys27 (Fig. 4).
3) F12 consists of two low affinity sites for Ca^{2+} and F34 two high affinity sites (Fig. 2).
4) F12 is equivalent to N-domain of calmodulin and F34 to C-domain.

Recent NMR studies on proteolytic fragments of calmodulin demonstrated that the tertiary structures of F12 and F34 were almost the same as those of corresponding N-domain and C-domain in the intact calmodulin, respectively, in the absence and presence of Ca^{2+} (18). This result indicates that calmodulin is composed of two large domains whose tertiary structures are rather independent of each other.

Saturation of C-domain by 2 mol of Ca^{2+} induces a remarkable conformational change on calmodulin (5,19,20). Increase in the hydrophobic region of calmodulin results from this conformational change (21), and the hydrophobic interaction between calmodulin and enzymes may play a part in their combination.

For the activation of enzymes, it is necessary to add more than 2 mol of Ca^{2+} to calmodulin. Tertiary structures of N-domain should be identical among calmodulins isolated from various animals because the primary structures are the same. An additional 1 or 2 mol of Ca^{2+} binds to N-domain and then the enzyme becomes active in association with the Ca^{2+}-bound N-domain of calmodulin. In the active state, the N-domain may be bound to a certain region of the enzyme. Since the N-domain structure is unvarying among animal calmodulins, the structure of enzymes matched to N-domain may also be identical. It is of interest to learn whether calmodulin-dependent enzymes really contain a common structure in their active site. It is also worthwhile noting that the N-domain alone (F12) cannot activate enzymes even in the presence of Ca^{2+} (22).

In brief, N-domain and C-domain of calmodulin may have different functions, i.e., activation and combination, respectively. The manner of enzyme recognition of the C-domain may vary but there may be a common enzyme site relative to the N-domain.

REFERENCES

1. Vanaman, T. C., Sharief, F., and Watterson, D. M., in
    "Calcium Binding Protein and Calcium Function" (R. H.
    Wasserman, et al., eds.), p. 107. Elsevier, North
    Holland, Amsterdam, 1977.
2. Toda, H., Yazawa, M., Kondo, K., Honma, T., Narita, K.,
    and Yagi, K., J. Biochem. 90:1493 (1981).
3. Crouch, T. M., and Klee, C. B., Biochemistry 19:3692
    (1980).
4. Blumenthal, D. K., and Stull, J. T., Biochemistry 19:5608
    (1980).
5. Yagi, K., Matsuda, S., Nagamoto, H., Mikuni, T., and
    Yazawa, M., in "Calmodulin and Intracellular Ca^{2+}
    Receptors" (S. Kakiuchi, H. Hidaka, and A. R. Means,
    eds.), p. 75. Plenum Publishing Corp., New York, 1982.
6. Kilhoffer, M. C., Gerald, D., and Demaille, J. G., FEBS
    Lett. 120:99 (1980).
7. Wang, C. A., Aguaron, R. R., Leavis, P. C., and Gergely,
    J., Eur. J. Biochem. 124:7 (1982).
8. Wallace, R. W., Tallant, E. A., Dockter, M. E., and
    Cheung, W. Y., J. Biol. Chem. 257:1845 (1982).
9. Yazawa, M., Sakuma, M., and Yagi, K., J. Biochem. 87:1313
    (1980).
10. Drabikowski, W., Brzeska, H., and Venyaminov, S. Y., J.
    Biol. Chem. 257:11584 (1982).
11. Yoshida, M., Minowa, O., and Yagi, K., J. Biochem.
    94:1925 (1983).
12. Yazawa, M., Kawamura, E., Minowa, O., Yagi, K., Ikura,
    M., and Hikichi, K., J. Biochem. in press (1984).
13. Adair, G. S., J. Biol. Chem. 63:529 (1925).
14. Tanaka, T., and Yamaoka, K., in "Guide of the
    Microcomputer for Chemists" (in Japanese), p. 114.
    Nankodo, Tokyo, 1981.
15. Haiech, J., Klee, C. B., and Demaille, J. G.,
    Biochemistry 20:3890 (1981).
16. Minowa, O., Yoshida, M., and Yagi, K., (Submitted to J.
    Biochem.)(1984).
17. Potter, J. D., and Gergely, J., J. Biol. Chem. 250:4628
    (1975).
18. Ikura, M., Hiraoki, T., Hikichi, K., Minowa, O.,
    Yamaguchi, H., Yazawa, M., and Yagi, K., Biochemistry in
    press (1984).
19. Klee, C. B., Biochemistry 16:1017 (1977).
20. Ikura, M., Hiraoki, T., Hikichi, K., Mikuni, T., Yazawa,
    M., and Yagi, K., Biochemistry 22:2568 (1983).
21. Tanaka, T., and Hidaka, H., J. Biol. Chem. 255:11078
    (1980).

22. Perry, S. V., in "Muscle Contraction, Its Regulatory
     Mechanism" (S. Ebashi, K. Maruyama, and M. Endo, eds.),
     p. 207. Japan Sci. Soc. Press, Tokyo, 1980.

CALCINEURIN, A Ca^{2+} AND CALMODULIN-REGULATED PROTEIN PHOSPHATASE

Claude B. Klee
Allan S. Manalan
Marie H. Krinks

Laboratory of Biochemistry
National Cancer Institute
National Institutes of Health
Bethesda, Maryland

Alastair Aitken[1]
Philip Cohen

Department of Biochemistry
University of Dundee,
Scotland

I. INTRODUCTION

Several years ago we purified one of the major calmodulin-binding proteins of brain and called it calcineurin because of its ability to bind Ca^{2+} and its specific distribution in tissues of neural origin (1,2). This protein, first detected as a heat-labile inhibitor of the calmodulin stimulation of cyclic nucleotide phosphodiesterase, was subsequently shown to be a potent and specific inhibitor of other calmodulin actions (3-7). The discovery by Stewart et al. (8) of a calmodulin-regulated protein phosphatase (protein phosphatase 2B) with a subunit composition similar to that of calcineurin led

---

[1]Present address: Department of Pharmaceutical Chemistry, School of Pharmacy, University of London, London WC1N-1AX, England.

CALCIUM REGULATION
IN BIOLOGICAL SYSTEMS

to the demonstration that calcineurin is a protein phosphatase under the dual control of Ca^{2+} and calmodulin (9).

II. PHYSICAL AND CHEMICAL PROPERTIES OF CALCINEURIN

Calcineurin is a heterodimer composed of a large 61,000 dalton subunit (calcineurin A) and a small 19,000 dalton subunit (calcineurin B)(1,5,10). The two subunits interact with each other in the absence of divalent metal ions to form an 80,000 Mr protein (1,4). The physical properties of calcineurin are summarized in Table I.

Calcineurin binds 3-4 mol of Ca^{2+} with high affinity ($K_{diss} \leq 10^{-6}$ M) in the presence of physiological concentrations of Mg^{2+} and K^+ (1). Ca^{2+} binding is accompanied by a conformational change which affects the environment of the aromatic residues of the protein. Because the electrophoretic migration of calcineurin B in SDS gels is affected by the presence of Ca^{2+} or EGTA (apparent Mr of 15,000 and 16,000 respectively) it was proposed to be the Ca^{2+} binding subunit. The amino acid sequence of calcineurin B, a 168 residue polypeptide, has been determined by Aitken et al. (11) and revealed the existence of four putative "EF-hand" Ca^{2+} binding-loops analogous to those of the other intracellular Ca^{2+}-binding proteins. In contrast to the high degree of homology between the Ca^{2+} loops of calcineurin B and those of calmodulin, there is only 35% homology between the overall sequences of the two proteins. Protein secondary structure predictions suggest that the peptide segment between the first two Ca^{2+} sites has a different conformation in the two proteins. The NH_2 and COOH terminal tails of calcineurin B as well as the connecting peptide between Site III and IV are larger than those of calmodulin. In addition, calcineurin B has an amino terminal glycyl residue blocked with myristic acid, which contributes to the hydrophobic character of this protein (12). These differences may explain why the two proteins are not functionally cross-reacting. Calcineurin B can neither replace calmodulin in its activation of phosphodiesterase or calcineurin nor inhibit calmodulin stimulation of the two enzymes. Conversely, calmodulin does not replace calcineurin B in our attempts to reconstitute calcineurin from its isolated components.

Calcineurin A is the calmodulin binding subunit of calcineurin. It binds one mol of calmodulin per mol in the presence of Ca^{2+} but not in its absence. It therefore contains two protein interaction sites: one for calcineurin B, and one for calmodulin. As indicated above these interaction domains are highly specific for their respective protein ligands. Limited proteolysis of calcineurin A with trypsin also re-

TABLE I.   Physical and Chemical Properties of Calcineurin

	Calcineurin		Trypsin-Calcineurin	
	EGTA	$Ca^{2+} \cdot CaM$	EGTA	$Ca^{2+} \cdot CaM$
$M_r{}^a$	80,000	95,000		
$s_{20,w}(S)^b$	4.5	5.0	4.3	4.3
Subunit composition				
A (61K)	A.B	CaM.A.B	A'.B	A'.B
A' (45K)				
B (19K)				
K_{CaM} (M^{-1})	$<10^{5c}$	3×10^{8d}		$<10^{5c}$
Phosphatase[e] (nmol/min/mg)	0.4	2.2	3.1	1.6

[a]M_r was determined by cross-linking with dimethyl-suberimidate.

[b]Sedimentation coefficients and subunit composition determined by glycerol gradient centrifugation (13).

[c]No complex of calcineurin and calmodulin was observed during glycerol gradient centrifugation of calcineurin (10^{-6}M) in the presence of 7.5×10^{-7} M calmodulin (13).

[d]As determined in ref. 4.

[e]As determined in ref. 13 using smooth muscle myosin light chains (10^{-6} M).

(Taken from Ref. 30).

vealed important differences between the two protein binding domains (13). Whereas the calcineurin B site is resistant to trypsin, the calmodulin-binding domain is highly susceptible to limited proteolysis. In the absence of calmodulin trypsin rapidly degraded calcineurin A to a 45,000 dalton fragment, which does not bind calmodulin, as well as small peptides. The presence of calmodulin protects calcineurin A against proteolysis. The digestion proceeds more slowly, intermediate size polypeptides (57,000, 55,000, 54,000 and 46,000 Mr) which still bind calmodulin are produced; but upon prolonged digestion a 45,000 Mr fragment is also generated. Calmodulin and calcineurin B are not significantly degraded by trypsin under these conditions.

III. CALCINEURIN IS A MAJOR CALMODULIN BINDING PROTEIN IN BRAIN

When brain proteins are resolved by SDS gel electrophoresis, three major calmodulin-binding proteins are detected in crude extracts by the gel overlay method using $[^{125}I]$-calmodulin(Fig. 1). The 240,000 Mr polypeptide is the large subunit of an actin-binding, spectrin-like, protein now known as fodrin or calspectin (14-18). The subunit size of the 50,000 Mr component may correspond to that of the multifunctional, calmodulin-stimulated, protein kinase(s) (19-21). The 61,000 Mr polypeptide has been identified as the large subunit of calcineurin by Western blot analyses with anti-calcineurin antibodies. Quantitative analysis of immunoblots of crude brain extracts revealed that calcineurin accounts for most of the 61,000 dalton protein detected by the gel overlay method. Calcineurin levels in brain could be as high as 600-800 mg per kg (10^{-5} M). Since the Western blots detect both the small and the large subunits of calcineurin we were able to show that, even in crude extracts, the two subunits of calcineurin are present in a one-to-one ratio.

Whereas fodrin, a membrane-associated protein, is solubilized preferentially at high ionic strength, the 50,000 Mr protein is soluble only in the presence of detergents. The latter protein is therefore likely to be an integral membrane protein. Calcineurin, on the other hand, is partially soluble (30%) in low or high ionic strength buffers. Addition of detergent to the extraction medium releases another 40% of the calcineurin, but 30% of the protein appears to be resistant to these extraction procedures. Thus calcineurin, in contrast to the other calmodulin-binding proteins, appears to have a heterogenous subcellular distribution in brain. It could be partitioned between the soluble, membranous and cytoskeletal compartments of the cell.

IV. CALCINEURIN IS A PROTEIN PHOSPHATASE

Protein phosphatase activity measured by the Ca^{2+}-dependent dephosphorylation of histones or p-nitrophenylphosphate can be detected in brain homogenates and is only partially solubilized in the absence of detergents. In crude fractions a precise correlation between calcineurin levels and Ca^{2+}-dependent protein phosphatase activity is prevented by the presence of other phosphatases and the large amount of endogenous substrates which act as apparent inhibitors. However, during subsequent purification steps, calmodulin-stimulated protein phosphatase and calcineurin, assayed by the gel overlay method, copurify as illustrated in Fig. 2 (22). Additional fractionation procedures such as hydroxylapatite

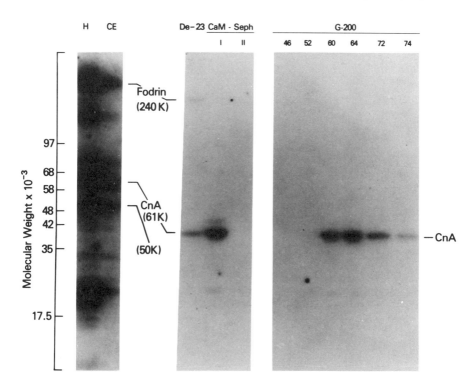

FIGURE 1. Purification of bovine brain calcineurin. Calcineurin was analyzed by the gel overlay method throughout the purification procedure (22). H, homogenate; CE, crude extract; DE 23, pooled fraction after DE 23 cellulose chromatography; CaM–Seph, material eluted with EGTA from the calmodulin–Sepharose affinity column. (I, first; II, second passage through the column); G-200, fractions from the Sephadex G-200 gel filtration. The migration and Mr of fodrin, calcineurin A and the 50 K protein are indicated on the figure.

chromatography (22), glycerol gradient centrifugation (13,23), gel electrophoresis (23), and chromatofocusing (9) also failed to resolve calcineurin from the phosphatase activity. Recently, Tonks and Cohen have demonstrated the Ca^{2+}-dependent interaction of calcineurin with thiophosphorylated light chains coupled to Sepharose, providing further evidence that calcineurin is indeed a protein phosphatase (24). The Ca^{2+}-dependent interaction of calcineurin with radiolabeled thiophosphorylated myosin light chains has also been detected by cross-linking with dimethylsuberimidate as illustrated in Fig. 3. A cross-linked, radioactive polypeptide with a Mr of

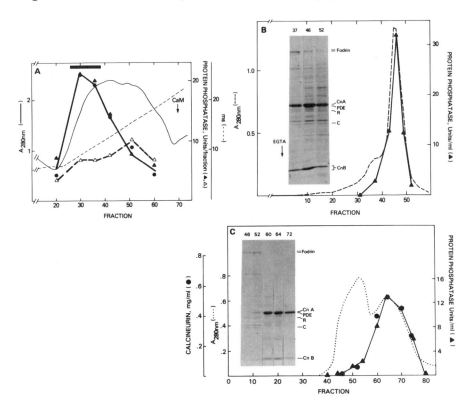

FIGURE 2. Purification of bovine brain calcineurin according to ref. 22. A, DE 23 chromatography (23); B, calmodulin Sepharose affinity chromatography; C, Sephadex G-200 gel filtration. Calcineurin was assayed by the gel overlay method (●); protein phosphatase by dephosphorylation of [^{32}P] labeled myosin light chains (A) and histones (B, C) in the presence (▲) or absence (△) of calmodulin. Inset: SDS gel electrophoretic pattern of the fractions shown on the figure.

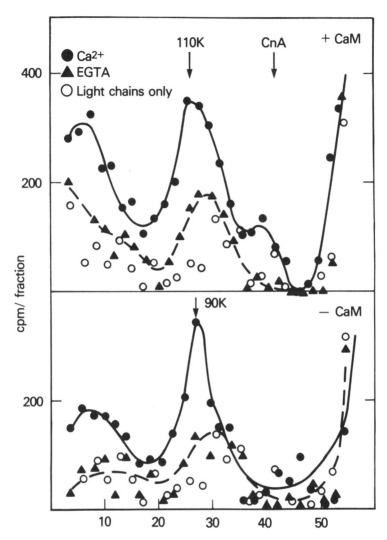

FIGURE 3. Cross-linking of calcineurin with [^{35}S]-thiophosphorylated myosin light chains. Cross-linking with dimethylsuberimidate was performed as described in ref. 4 in the presence or absence of 4 M calmodulin as shown on the figure. Calcineurin was 3.5 M and thiophosphorylated light chains were 6.5 M; when present CaCl$_2$ was 1.5 mM or EGTA 3 mM. The migration of calcineurin A and the Mr of the radioactive peaks are indicated on the figure.

Cross-linked polypeptides were resolved by SDS gel electrophoresis. Gels were cut in 1 mm slices. Radioactivity in gel slices is plotted as a function of slice number. The tracking dye was at slice 90.

90,000 corresponds to a 1:1:1 complex of calcineurin A, calcineurin B and myosin light chain. In the presence of calmodulin, which also interacts with the enzyme, a quaternary complex is formed with an apparent Mr of 110,000. The Ca^{2+}-dependent interaction reflects the requirement for Ca^{2+} binding to calcineurin B to increase the affinity of the substrate for the enzyme (24). Ca^{2+} binding to myosin light chains could also affect the interaction. Limited proteolysis of calcineurin with trypsin has also been used to corroborate protein phosphatase activity of calcineurin (13). A large increase in phosphatase activity (measured in the presence of EGTA) accompanies the proteolytic cleavage of calcineurin A. The proteolyzed Ca^{2+}-independent enzyme, which does not interact with calmodulin, sediments with a slightly lower sedimentation coefficient (4.3S) than the native enzyme (4.5S). Trypsin treated calcineurin is a heterodimer of the 45,000 dalton proteolytic product of calcineurin A and calcineurin B (Table I). In the presence of calmodulin, proteolysis proceeds more slowly (as indicated above); similarly, the activation of the enzyme and concomitant loss of calmodulin stimulation occur at a very slow rate. A schematic representation of the activation of calcineurin by calmodulin and limited proteolysis is illustrated in Fig. 4.

All of these experiments demonstrate that calcineurin is a protein phosphatase regulated by Ca^{2+} in two ways. The enzymatic activity is almost entirely dependent upon Ca^{2+} binding to calcineurin B. An additional 5- to 10-fold stimulation the enzyme follows the Ca^{2+}-dependent binding of one mol of calmodulin per mol of calcineurin (9). This calmodulin stimulation affects the V_{max} of the enzyme and has no significant effect on the Km value for the substrate. In contrast to some other protein phosphatases which have a broad specificity towards their substrates, calcineurin exhibits a high degree of substrate specificity (9,25). The only proteins which are known to be dephosphorylated at a fast rate (0.5 to 2 $\mu mol/min/mg$) are the α-subunit of phosphorylase kinase, inhibitor-1 of protein phosphatase and the type II regulatory subunit of cAMP-dependent protein kinase (9,22,26). Other substrates such as myosin light chains from skeletal and smooth muscles, and the protein substrate of cyclic GMP dependent protein kinase (G protein) are dephosphorylated more slowly (0.1 - 0.5 $\mu mol/min/mg$) (9,22,27). Calcineurin can also dephosphorylate casein, histones VS and IIa (but at much reduced rates) and model substrates such as phosphotyrosine and p-nitrophenylphosphate (28,29). Phosphotyrosine in proteins, however, is a poor substrate[1]. Like that of other

---

[1]D. Werth, unpublished results.

protein phosphatases, the enzymatic activity of calcineurin is
stimulated by other divalent metal ions which appear to
interact with the catalytic unit of the enzyme. Mn^{2+} and
Ni^{2+} have been reported to have a pronounced stimulatory
effect particularly on the p-nitrophenylphosphatase activity
of the enzyme (28,29).

Protein phosphorylation and dephosphorylation must play
important and unique roles in the brain. The tissue is an
extremely rich source of the enzymes of cAMP metabolism and of
protein kinases. The demonstration that a major brain protein, calcineurin, is a protein phosphatase identifies an
important component of this regulatory system.

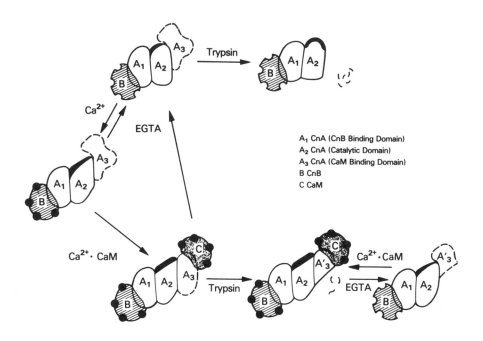

FIGURE 4. Schematic representation of the activation of
calcineurin by Ca^{2+}, Ca^{2+}-CaM and trypsin. A_2, A_1, A_3 are the
catalytic, calcineurin B, and calmodulin-binding domains of
calcineurin A respectively. B is calcineurin B, C is calmodulin. The semi-circles represent the Ca^{2+} binding sites in the
free state and the filled circles in the liganded state. The
catalytic site on calcineurin A is shown by the darkened area
(From ref. 30).

REFERENCES

1. Klee, C. B., Crouch, T. H., and Krinks, M. H., Proc.
    Natl. Acad. Sci. USA 76:6270 (1980).
2. Wallace, R. W., Tallant, E. A., and Cheung, W. Y.,
    Biochemistry 19:1831 (1980).
3. Wang, J. H., and Desai, R., J. Biol. Chem. 252:4175
    (1977).
4. Klee, C. B., and Krinks, M. H., Biochemistry 17:120
    (1978).
5. Wallace, R. W., Lynch, T. J., Tallant, E. A., and Cheung,
    W. Y., J. Biol. Chem. 254:377 (1979).
6. Larsen, F. L., Raess, B. U., Hinds, T. R., and Vincenzi,
    F. F., J. Supramol. Structure 9:269 (1978).
7. Cohen, P., Picton, C., and Klee, C. B., FEBS Lett. 104:25
    (1979).
8. Stewart, A. A., Ingebritsen, T. S., and Cohen, P., Eur.
    J. Biochem. 132:289 (1983).
9. Stewart, A. A., Ingebritsen, T. S., Manalan, A., Klee,
    C. B., and Cohen, P., FEBS Lett. 137:80 (1982).
10. Sharma, R. K., Desai, R., Waisman, D. M., and Wang, J.
    H., J. Biol. Chem. 254:4276 (1979).
11. Aitken, A., Klee, C. B., Stewart, A. A., Tonks, N. K.,
    and Cohen, P., in "Calcium-Binding Proteins" (B.
    deBernard et al., eds.), p.113, Elsevier North Holland,
    Amsterdam, 1983.
12. Aitken, A., Cohen, P., Santikarn, S., Williams, D. H.,
    Calder, A. G., Smith, A., and Klee, C. B., FEBS Lett.
    150:314 (1982).
13. Manalan, A. S., and Klee, C. B., Proc. Natl. Acad. Sci.
    USA 80:4291 (1983).
14. Davies, P. J. A., and Klee, C. B., Biochem. Int. 3:203
    (1981).
15. Levine, J., and Willard, M., J. Cell Biol. 90:631 (1981).
16. Kakiuchi, S., Sobue, K., and Fujita, M., FEBS Lett.
    132:144 (1981).
17. Glenney, J. R., Glenney, P., and Weber, K., Proc. Natl.
    Acad. Sci. USA 79:4002 (1982).
18. Kakiuchi, S., Neurochem. Int. 5:159 (1983).
19. Fukunaga, K., Yamamoto, H., Matsui, K., Higashi, K., and
    Miyamoto, E., J. Neurochem. 132:15 (1982).
20. Yamauchi, T., and Fujisawa, H., Eur. J. Biochem. 132:15
    (1983).
21. Kennedy, M. B., McGuiness, T., and Greengard, P., J.
    Neurosci. 3:818 (1983).
22. Klee, C. B., Krinks, M. H., Manalan, A. S., Cohen, P.,
    and Stewart, A. A., Meth. Enzymol. 102:227 (1983).
23. Yang, S. -D., Tallant, E. A., and Cheung, W. Y., Biochem.

Biophys. Res. Commun. 106:1419 (1982).
24.   Tonks, N. K., and Cohen, P., Biochim. Biophys. Acta
      747:191 (1983).
25.   Ingebritsen, T. S., and Cohen, P., Science 221:331
      (1983).
26.   Blumenthal, D. K., and Krebs, E. G., Biophys. J. 41:409a
      (1983).
27.   King, M. M., Huang, C. Y., Chock, P. B., Nairn, A. C.,
      Hemmings, H. C., Jr., Chan, K. -F. J., and Greengard, P.,
      Fed. Proc. Am. Soc. Exp. Biol. 42:1801 (1983).
28.   Pallen, C. J., and Wang, J. H., J. Biol. Chem. 258:8550
      (1983).
29.   King, M. M., and Huang, C. Y., Biochem. Biophys. Res.
      Commun. 114:955 (1983).
30.   Klee, C. B., Krinks, M. H., and Manalan, A. S., in
      "Calcium Binding Proteins" (B. deBernard et al., eds.)
      p.103, Elsevier North Holland, Amsterdam, 1983.

PHOSPHORYLATION OF SMOOTH MUSCLE MYOSIN[1]

David. J. Hartshorne
Mitsuo Ikebe

Muscle Biology Group
Agricultural Sciences Building
University of Arizona
Tucson, Arizona

I. INTRODUCTION

A distinctive feature of the smooth muscle contractile apparatus is that regulation is manifest as an activation of contractile activity in the presence of Ca^{2+}, as opposed to a depression of activity in the absence of Ca^{2+} for the skeletal muscle system (1). This concept is accepted as representing the fundamental requirement for regulation in smooth muscle but the nature, or identity, of the activator remains controversial.

The most popular theory is that the activation of contractile activity is based on the phosphorylation-dephosphorylation of the two 20,000-dalton light chains of the myosin molecule. This theory originated with the report by Sobieszek (2) who showed that phosphorylation of myosin was accompanied by an increase in the level of actin-activated ATPase activity. Subsequently a considerable body of evidence has been accumulated. The most basic interpretation is that phosphorylation fully activates the contractile apparatus and dephosphorylation inactivates the system. With this concept there is very little opportunity for the modulation of contractile response, unless singly- and doubly-phosphorylated myosin have different properties, and this situation obviously is oversimplified.

---

[1]This work was supported by grants HL 23615 and HL 20984 from the National Institutes of Health.

41

In order to account for the variety and complexity of the contractile responses in smooth muscle it seems that other factors need to be implicated. For example, it was shown by Adelstein and coworkers (4,5) that the myosin light chain kinase (MLCK) molecule can be phosphorylated by the cAMP-dependent protein kinase and that phosphorylation at a specific site results in a decrease in the affinity of the enzyme for calmodulin. Under conditions where the concentration of the Ca^{2+}-calmodulin complex is limiting this would facilitate relaxation. Evidence cited in favor of an additional mechanism also is given in the experiments of Dillon et al. (6) and Chatterjee and Murphy (7). They found that the load-bearing capacity of strips of carotid artery was maintained despite a reduction in the extent of myosin phosphorylation. Their interpretation of this phenomenon was that myosin phosphorylation determines the rate of cross bridge cycling (which is fully consistent with the biochemical evidence) but that an additional component is responsible for the maintenance of tension or load-bearing capacity. It was suggested by these authors and others (8,9) that under certain conditions non-cycling cross bridges could form which would effectively fix the muscle at a given load and maintain tension at a reduced rate of ATP hydrolysis. Since these non-cycling cross bridges are presumably released when the muscle relaxes it is argued that the attachment-detachment process is Ca^{2+}-dependent and therefore would implicate an additional mechanism. An alternative explanation might be that myosin phosphorylation could control cross bridge kinetics, but there is no evidence to support this idea.

A critical component of the phosphorylation scheme is the dephosphorylation reaction and this is an area with obvious deficiencies. The identity of the phosphatase(s) has not been established and it is not known if the phosphatase is subject to regulation. It is generally assumed that the phosphatase is active both in the presence and absence of Ca^{2+} but its effect is manifest only in the absence of Ca^{2+} and a preference for the latter would be expected.

Other mechanisms which might operate in conjunction with myosin phosphorylation include the thin filament system outlined by Walters and Marston (10) and the direct binding of Ca^{2+} to myosin proposed by Chacko and Rosenfeld (11). A mechanism proposed as an alternative to myosin phosphorylation is the leiotonin system (12). Over the past few years the roles and in vivo relevance of leiotonin and of phosphorylation have been controversial and the situation still is not resolved. (For a further discussion on leiotonin see Prof. Ebashi's article in this volume.)

In spite of the above deficiencies and uncertainties there is considerable evidence to suggest that phosphorylation of myosin is at least a component of the regulatory system in smooth muscle. The current requirement is to evaluate the exact role of phosphorylation and in particular to identify any other complementary, or alternative systems. To this end we have been analyzing in vitro the phosphorylation and dephosphorylation reactions and have attempted to define some of the consequences of phosphorylation on the properties and conformation of smooth muscle myosin. Some of these results are presented below.

II. EFFECT OF PHOSPHORYLATION ON ATPASE ACTIVITY

The observation which led to the formulation of the phosphorylation theory was that the Mg^{2+}-ATPase activity of gizzard actomyosin increased as the level of myosin phosphorylation increased (2). In subsequent studies using a variety of experimental systems (reviews 1,3) the positive correlation between phosphorylation and actin-activated ATPase activity was confirmed and a more recent concern centered on the effects of phosphorylation of the two myosin light chains each associated with one of the two myosin heads. For example, does phosphorylation of one light chain of myosin molecule activate a single head or both heads, or is phosphorylation of both sites required for ATPase activation?

With such considerations in mind Persechini and Hartshorne (13) measured the actin-activated ATPase activity of myosin which was phosphorylated to varying degrees. Phosphorylation of up to one site per molecule produced only a slight activation, whereas, phosphorylation of the second site was accompanied by a marked increase in ATPase activity. Our explanation of this behavior was that phosphorylation of both heads of the myosin molecule is required for activation of ATPase activity and this suggested some form of cooperativity between the two myosin heads. Similar relationships between phosphorylation and ATPase activity have since been reported (14,15) although in the later study (15) the level of ATPase activity was considerably higher than in the other reports. Although this pattern appears valid for in vitro studies the requirement for double phosphorylation has not been shown in either intact or skinned smooth muscle fibers, and this is obviously a critical point to establish. Another consideration is that although it seems reasonable to assume that both myosin heads are activated via double phosphorylation it is also possible that only one head is activated.

III. PHOSPHORYLATION–DEPHOSPHORYLATION REACTION

Are the two 20,000-dalton light chains of myosin equivalent as substrates for the myosin light chain kinase? The first clue to their nonequivalence was obtained in the study discussed above (13) on the phosphorylation-dependence of ATPase activity. If double phosphorylation of myosin is required for actin activation of ATPase activity and if both light chains are equivalent substrates (i.e., to generate random phosphorylation) then the increase in ATPase activity would follow the square of the fractional phosphorylation, i.e., at 40% total phosphorylation 16% of the myosin molecules would be doubly phosphorylated and activated by actin. The curve relating ATPase activity and random phosphorylation can therefore be constructed and compared to the actual data. It was found (13,14) that the relationship between phosphorylation and ATPase activity did not fit the random curve but showed a more exaggerated dependence on phosphorylation. At lower levels of phosphorylation it was particularly noticeable that the ATPase activity was lower than expected from random phosphorylation. This suggested that myosin at relatively low ionic strength is phosphorylated in a sequential manner, one light chain of myosin being a preferred substrate to the other light chain. The same conclusion was derived from experiments done at different concentrations of MLCK, which showed essentially two classes of substrate for the phosphorylation reaction (13) and also from time courses of phosphorylation (16). An interesting point is that once the light chains are removed from the myosin molecule only one class of substrate is observed, which suggests that the nonidentity of phosphorylation sites is not due to chemical inhomogeneity but might be related to the location or structure of the light chains in the native molecule. However, even if the sequential phosphorylation is imposed by the location or interactions of the light chains in native myosin it is not an inherent property of myosin under all conditions. Heavy meromyosin (14,17) and myosin at high ionic strength (17), both show random phosphorylation and therefore whatever factor generates the ordered reaction it may or may not be expressed.

There are two simple possibilities to explain sequential, or ordered phosphorylation. The first is the result of negative cooperativity between the light chains. The phosphorylation of one light chain would reduce the ability of the second light chain to be phosphorylated. The other explanation, termed preexisting asymmetry, simply assumes that prior to phosphorylation each light chain exists in a different state and that each state has a distinct reactivity as a substrate for the kinase. The negative cooperative and preexisting asymmetry models are illustrated in a diagrammatic form in Fig. 1. It is rather difficult to distinguish between these two possibilities but our preference based on kinetic analyses of the substrate concentration dependence favors the preexisting asymmetry model (16).

The pathway of dephosphorylation has not been studied as extensively as the phosphorylation reaction. It was suggested that the dephosphorylation of heavy meromyosin followed a

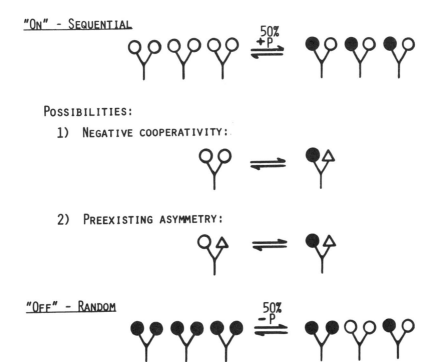

FIGURE 1. Diagrammatic representation of the mechanisms of phosphorylation and dephosphorylation. Circles and triangles represent myosin heads; open and closed symbols represent dephosphorylated and phosphorylated heads, respectively. "On" reaction indicates the sequence of phosphorylation when half of the total light chains are phosphorylated. Negative cooperativity model suggests that phosphorylation of one head alters the conformation of the second head (i.e., the dephosphorylated head). Preexisting asymmetry model suggests that the two heads of dephosphorylated myosin are different and exist in rapidly reacting (o) and slowly reacting (Δ) states. "Off" reaction indicates the random mechanism of dephosphorylation in going from fully phosphorylated myosin to myosin in which half of the light chains are phosphorylated.

course consistent with positive cooperativity (18). In our
laboratory, however, we have found that the dephosphorylation
of gizzard myosin occurs in a random manner. This is depicted
diagrammatically in Fig. 1 and the experimental data are shown
in Fig. 2. In Fig. 2A the time course of dephosphorylation is
shown and as indicated in the inset follows a single exponential. The actin-activated ATPase activity shown in Fig. 2B,
also is consistent with random dephosphorylation since the
data points follow closely the predicted square of the fractional phosphorylation relationship (solid line).

The conventional view, or at least that consistent with
the phosphorylation theory, is that the dephosphorylation of
myosin is a prerequisite for relaxation. This raises the
question of whether the phosphatase prefers the attached or
detached cross bridge. One approach to this problem is to
determine the effect of actin on the in vitro dephosphorylation of myosin and this is shown in Fig. 2A. Clearly, actin

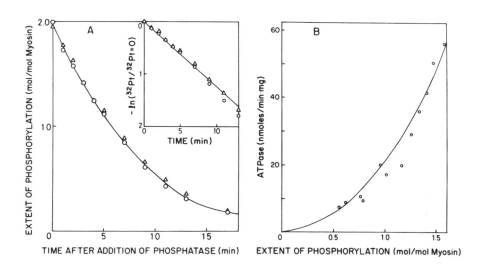

FIGURE 2. Dephosphorylation of gizzard myosin. A) Time
course of dephosphorylation in the absence (o) and presence
(△) of 1 mg/ml F-actin. Inset: semi-log plot. B) Relationship between phosphorylation level and ATPase during dephosphorylation. Phosphorylation of turkey gizzard myosin was
obtained by the addition of $[\gamma-^{32}P]ATP$ (1 mM) to: 1 mg/ml
myosin, 7.5 μg/ml MLCK, 5 μg/ml calmodulin, 8 mM $MgCl_2$, 75 mM
KCl, 0.1 mM $CaCl_2$, 25 mM Tris-HCl (pH 7.5). After 10 min
phosphatase fraction, 1 mg/ml F-actin and EGTA (2 mM) were
added and samples were taken at different time intervals to
determine the time course and ATPase-dependence with
dephosphorylation.

(at approximately 11 fold molar excess over myosin) has no detectable effect on the dephosphorylation rate, even at low levels of phosphorylation where one might expect slower ATP hydrolysis.

IV. EFFECTS OF PHOSPHORYLATION ON THE PROPERTIES OF MYOSIN

Since the phosphorylation of smooth muscle myosin allows subsequent activation by actin of Mg^{2+}-ATPase activity one would expect some molecular alteration to be induced by phosphorylation. Although the phosphorylation-dependent molecular changes are not defined there are some interesting recent observations which may help in understanding the molecular mechanism. Suzuki et al. (19) showed that filaments of dephosphorylated myosin in 0.15 M KCl were disassembled by ATP and on ultracentrifugation formed a major component of approximately 10S. However, at higher ionic strengths only a 6S component was detected both in the absence and presence of ATP. At this time it was suggested (19) that the 10S conformation reflected a myosin dimer, and the 6S form the myosin monomer. It was later shown (20) that in fact both the 10S and 6S forms were monomeric myosin and that the increase in sedimentation coefficient resulted from a decrease in the radius of gyration. This extensive change in hydrodynamic properties was visualized by electron microscopy for gizzard (21,22), vascular muscle (23) and thymus myosin (22). It was found that the 10S component formed a looped structure in which the tail of the myosin molecule is bent over towards the head region. In contrast the 6S component remained in the extended, more asymmetric form. It was also suggested that the transition from 6S to 10S was favored by dephosphorylation (22,23).

We have also been studying this transition by monitoring the viscosity of myosin and have been particularly interested in the effects of phosphorylation (24). In the presence of Mg^{2+}-ATP the 6S to 10S transition is favored by decreasing ionic strength and by dephosphorylation. For dephosphorylated myosin the relative viscosity, η_{rel} ($\eta_{protein}$/ $\eta_{solvent}$) decreases markedly at concentrations of KCl of < 0.35 M (Fig. 3A). In contrast η_{rel} of phosphorylated myosin is reduced only at lower ionic strengths, at less than approximately 0.2 M. These experiments were done with 1 mM ATP and 1 or 2 mM $MgCl_2$ (total concentrations). At higher concentrations of $MgCl_2$ (e.g., 10 mM concentration) aggregation of phosphorylated myosin may occur before any reduction in viscosity is observed (24). Under usual conditions ATP facilitates the conformational transition, however ATP is not obligatory and in Fig. 3A it is shown that dephosphorylated myosin in the absence of ATP at lower ionic strengths undergoes a partial transformation to a lower viscosity form.

Sedimentation velocity experiments were carried out under a variety of solvent conditions to correlate the "high" and "low" viscosity forms to the 6S and 10S species, respectively. Some examples are shown in the inset of Fig. 3A. In the upper

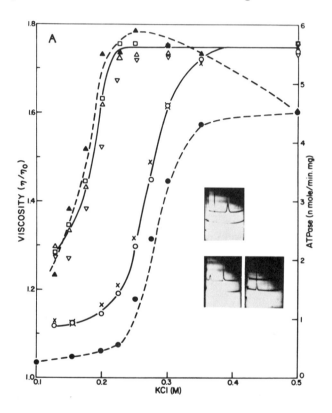

FIGURE 3A. KCl-dependence of Mg^{2+}-ATPase, viscosity and sedimentation patterns of phosphorylated and dephosphorylated gizzard myosin at 1 and 2 mM $MgCl_2$. Viscosity data: Dephosphorylated myosin, 1 mM ATP and 1 mM (o) or 2 mM $MgCl_2$ (X); dephosphorylated myosin minus ATP and 1 mM $MgCl_2$ (□); phosphorylated myosin, 1 mM ATP and 1 mM (△) or 2 mM $MgCl_2$ (▽). ATPase activity in 1 mM $MgCl_2$ shown for phosphorylated (▲) and dephosphorylated (●) myosin. Sedimentation patterns in 1 mM ATP and 1 mM $MgCl_2$ shown in insets, top: dephosphorylated myosin in 0.15 M KCl (upper) and 0.35 M KCl (lower) 32 min after reaching speed of 60,000 rpm, and bottom: phosphorylated myosin in 0.125 M KCl (upper) and 0.25 M KCl (lower) 1 min and 36 min after reaching speed of 60,000 rpm.

frame are shown the sedimentation patterns of dephosphorylated myosin in 0.15 and 0.35 M KCl. At both ionic strengths only one component is detectable and these are consistent with the 10S species at the lower ionic strength and the 6S species at the higher ionic strength. The lower frames show the sedimentation patterns at different times for phosphorylated myosin in 0.125 and 0.25 M KCl. At the lower ionic strength two sedimenting components are detected, representing the 10S species and myosin polymer; whereas at the higher ionic strength only the 6S species is observed.

In the presence of Ca^{2+}-ATP the viscosity transition is also observed (Fig. 3B). The viscosity of phosphorylated

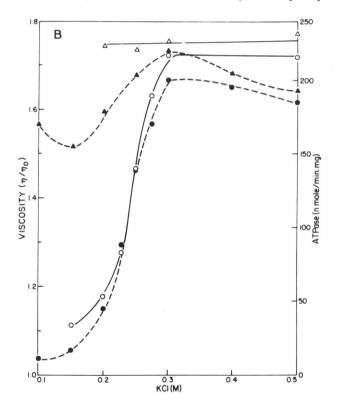

FIGURE 3B. KCl-dependence of Ca^{2+}-ATPase and viscosity for phosphorylated and dephosphorylated myosin at 7 mM $CaCl_2$. Myosin was phosphorylated and dialyzed versus 0.5 M KCl, 30 mM Tris-HCl (pH 7.5), 0.2 mM dithiothreitol. Viscosity data: dephosphorylated myosin and 1 mM ATP (o); phosphorylated myosin and 1 mM ATP ( ). ATPase activity shown for dephosphorylated (•) and phosphorylated myosin (▲). Figures reproduced from ref. 24, with permission.

myosin remains constant over a range of KCl concentrations from 0.2 to 0.5 M in contrast to η_{rel} of dephosphorylated myosin which is reduced markedly below 0.3 M KCl.

The ATPase activities of myosin were measured under identical conditions used for the viscosity experiments (24). The Mg^{2+}-ATPase and Ca^{2+}-ATPase activities are shown in Fig. 3A and 3B, respectively. A striking correlation is observed between the ATPase activity and the conformational transition. For the Mg^{2+}-ATPase activity of dephosphorylated myosin the decrease occurs over the same range of ionic strength as shown for the viscosity decrease. For the phosphorylated myosin the decrease in ATPase activity and viscosity occurs at a lower ionic strength but again both properties are correlated. An important point to emphasize is that the Mg^{2+}-ATPase activity does not show an absolute dependence on the state of myosin phosphorylation, since the formation of the 10S species with phosphorylated myosin is accompanied by a reduction of ATPase activity (Fig. 3A). The actin-activated ATPase activity of phosphorylated myosin at low Mg^{2+} and KCl concentrations of approximately 100 mM (i.e., under conditions where myosin forms the 10S) is also low. For the Ca^{2+}-ATPase activity a similar dependence of enzymatic activity and myosin conformation is demonstrated. The K^+ EDTA-ATPase of gizzard myosin also showed a dependence on the myosin conformation (24). In an earlier study by Onishi et al. (25) the KCl-dependence of these three types of ATPase activities were noted, but at that time the correlation to conformation was not realized.

As mentioned above the transition from the folded to extended form of myosin is enhanced by phosphorylation providing that the solvent conditions are appropriate. For example in 0.2 M KCl, 10 mM $MgCl_2$ and 1 mM ATP dephosphorylated myosin exists predominantly in the 10S form and phosphorylated myosin in the 6S form. The phosphorylation-dependence of this transition is shown in Fig. 4. The relationship between η_{rel} and the level of myosin phosphorylation is not linear and the major viscosity changes are observed at higher phosphorylation levels. From these results it appears unlikely that the phosphorylation of one of the myosin heads can achieve the complete transition to 6S and the latter is obtained only after phosphorylation of both sites. However, a slight increase in η_{rel} is observed at 50% phosphorylation (approximately 25% of total viscosity change) and is not known whether this reflects a partial unfolding of the myosin molecule or a shift in the 10S-6S equilibrium.

In addition to the changes in enzymatic activity which characterized each of the two myosin conformations it was shown that the ATP-induced fluorescence of the 10S and 6S species were distinct (26). The ATP-induced fluorescence is approximately 109 and 114% of the intrinsic tryptophan

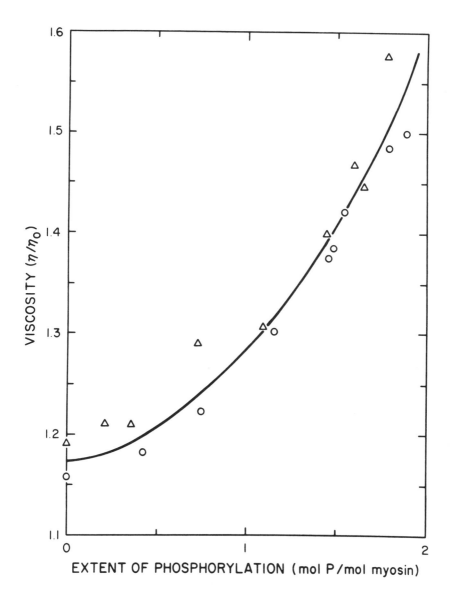

FIGURE 4.   Relationship between extent of myosin
phosphorylation   and   viscosity.   Varying   extents   of
phosphorylation obtained by varying kinase concentration and
time of incubation, reactions were stopped by addition of EGTA
(1 mM).   Phosphorylation carried out in either 75 mM KCl ($\triangle$)
or 0.2 M KCl (o).   Conditions for viscometry: 0.2 M KCl, 10
mM $MgCl_2$, 1 mM ATP, 1 mM EGTA, 30 mM Tris-HCl (pH 7.5).
Figure reproduced from ref. 24 with permission.

fluorescence in the absence of ATP for the 6S and 10S states of myosin, respectively. Under suitable solvent conditions the transition from 10S to 6S is driven by phosphorylation and if the ATP-induced fluorescence decrease is followed as a function of phosphorylation the relationship is virtually identical to that shown above (Fig. 4) for the viscosity measurements (26). This supports the contention that the fluorescence change is dictated by the myosin conformation.

It is known from earlier studies (27,28) that the addition of ATP to smooth muscle myosin enhances the tryptophan fluorescence, as it does with skeletal myosin. The amount of ATP required for the maximum steady-state fluorescence enhancement is approximately stoichiometric with the myosin heads. This would be compatible with the binding of ATP to the two ATP hydrolysis sites, since these are the only binding sites with the appropriate affinity (29). In addition it was shown previously that the viscosity transition also was effected by ATP concentrations stoichiometric with the myosin head concentration (24). Thus ATP binding at the active site facilitates a conformational change which is reflected by an alteration in the level of tryptophan fluorescence. Since the ATP-induced fluorescence enhancement is thought to be a component of the hydrolytic pathway, and since the enhancement occurs with either conformation it is reasonable to conclude that the tryptophan residues involved reflect changes occurring at the active sites. It is also reasonable to

Table I. Properties of 6S and 10S Smooth Muscle Myosin

Myosin	Shape	η_{rel}[a]	ATPase activities[b]			Fluorescence[c]
			Mg^{2+}	Ca^{2+}	K^+ EDTA	
6S	extended	~1.7	~4	~180	low	~109%
10S	looped	1.1-1.2	<1	~10	high	~114%

[a]The relative viscosity given for 2 mg/ml myosin.

[b]Numerical values expressed as nmoles P liberated/min/mg myosin. For the K^+ EDTA-ATPase activities because of the marked effect of varying K^+ concentrations it is not possible to obtain meaningful values for the 10S and 6S species.

[c]The fluorescence levels are expressed as a percentage of the intrinsic fluorescence of gizzard myosin obtained in the absence of ATP. Excitation 295 nm; emission 340 nm.

assume that these same residues are those that are sensitive
to the myosin conformation and following this line of
reasoning one can suggest that the active sites are affected
in some way by the myosin conformation. The notion that the
active sites are influenced by conformation obviously is a
very critical point and until this can be supported by direct
evidence it should be regarded only as speculation.

Before continuing it may be useful at this time to sum-
marize some of the characteristics of the 6S and 10S species
and these are given in Table I.

V. SHAPE-ACTIVITY RELATIONSHIP

The concept that is being developed is that interactions
involved in the shape changes of myosin alter enzymatic activity and could therefore be important in the regulation of
smooth muscle activity. A tentative suggestion is that the
10S species represents an "inactive" form and the 6S species
an "active" form and further that under physiological conditions the transition 10S to 6S (inactive to active) is
achieved by phosphorylation. The actin-activated ATPase
activity of myosin is obviously the relevant enzymatic property and evidence that this fits into the "shape" hypothesis
is only indirect and may be summarized as follows: the Mg^{2+}-,
Ca^{2+}- and K^+ EDTA-moderated ATPase activities show a marked
dependence on shape and when considered with the fluorescence
data would suggest that the active sites are influenced by
myosin conformation. In addition the phosphorylation-
dependence of the viscosity change and of the actin-activated
ATPase activity is nonlinear and in each case double
phosphorylation is required for the maximum effect. Finally,
the influence of varying Mg^{2+} concentrations (Ikebe and
Hartshorne, unpublished observations) is consistent with this
hypothesis. Increasing Mg^{2+} concentration causes: a) an
activation of actomyosin ATPase activity (both for phosphorylated and dephosphorylated myosin), b) a tendency to form the
6S species and, c) as shown in several earlier reports (30-34)
an increase in tension for skinned smooth muscle fibers but in
the absence of phosphorylation. The idea is that increasing
Mg^{2+} levels mimics, at least partially, the effects of
phosphorylation and causes the transition from the inactive to
the active species. This evidence is supportive of the shape-
activity hypothesis but is not conclusive and clearly one of
the priorities of future studies is to establish whether or
not such a relationship can exist under in vivo conditions.

Another point of considerable interest is whether the
shape transition involves a discrete intermediate confor-

mation. Obviously in going from the folded to extended form
intermediate shapes must be generated, but these may not be
stable and may exist only in the transitory state.   If,
however, a stable intermediate could be isolated it would be
important to define its biological properties.   For example,
is the ATPase activity high or low and does it bind to actin?
One objective for these studies would be to attempt a correlation between the noncycling cross bridges and myosin conformation.   It is possible that if an intermediate state does
exist its stability could be dependent on an additional regulatory mechanism, such as Ca^{2+} binding to myosin.

The shape of myosin may also be an important determinant
in the pattern of the phosphorylation, or dephosphorylation,
reactions.   At low ionic strength dephosphorylated myosin
exists as 10S and the subsequent phosphorylation reaction is
sequential. Dephosphorylated myosin at higher ionic strengths
forms 6S and the phosphorylation pattern is random (17).
Heavy meromyosin cannot form the 10S conformation, even at low
ionic strengths, and its phosphorylation is also random
(14,17).   Under usual conditions phosphorylated myosin favors
the 6S conformation and subsequent dephosphorylation is random.

A major reservation in accepting the "shape-activity"
hypothesis is that the bulk of the supportive experimental
data was obtained in vitro using monomeric myosin, and it is
now established that myosin in both relaxed and contracting
smooth muscles exists in the filamentous form (35).   It seems
unlikely that myosin packed into the thick filaments can form
the folded 10S conformation, but it is conceivable that inter-
molecular interaction (rather than intramolecular with monomeric myosin) might achieve the same effect.   It is to be
expected that the close association of molecules will alter
the properties of filamentous as compared to monomeric myosin,
but the extent of these modifications is not known.   Another
potential   problem   is   the   phosphorylation   of   filamentous
myosin. If myosin in the relaxed state is held in a fixed, or
rigid, conformation because of interactions equivalent to
those occurring in the 10S state, and if MLCK is bound to the
thin filament as suggested earlier (36) then there might be a
steric problem for the initial phosphorylation of the cross
bridge. Possibly the light chains of the cross bridges in
relaxed muscle could extend to within contact distance of the
thin filament-bound kinase, but details of geometry are not
available. Another possibility is that some other event
induces the thawing of the rigid cross bridge to approach more
closely to the MLCK. This could be analogous to a partial or
complete unfolding of the 10S state. Obviously if MLCK is not
restricted to the thin filament structure as suggested by
Sobue et al. (37) then these problems do not arise. Finally,

the properties of heavy meromyosin do not appear to fit into a simple 10S - 6S scheme. The actin-activated ATPase activity of heavy meromyosin is dependent on phosphorylation and although a slight ATP-induced conformational change may be detected (20) the 10S state cannot be formed since the interacting region in the tail of the myosin molecule is missing in heavy meromyosin. Thus for heavy meromyosin it is impossible that the regulation of ATPase activity can be attributed directly to the 10S - 6S transition. Possibly the critical events that modify enzymatic properties in myosin are more subtle and the gross conformational changes that occur (i.e., 10S to 6S) are merely coincidental to these other changes. The latter could still be present and effective in heavy meromyosin. But even if it is assumed that myosin and heavy meromyosin are equivalent with respect to the effects of phosphorylation they are not equivalent with respect to the effects of Mg^{2+}. With intact myosin increasing Mg^{2+} levels mimic to some degree the effects of phosphorylation, but are inhibitory with dephosphorylated heavy meromyosin. Why the two systems are not equivalent is not understood, and again the involvement of an additional factor may be indicated.

In summary we have presented some evidence in favor of a relationship between the enzymatic properties of myosin and its conformation. However, there are several aspects which are not understood and must be resolved before the idea can be accepted as anything better than a working hypothesis.

REFERENCES

1. Hartshorne, D. J., and Mrwa, U., Blood Vessels 19:1 (1982).
2. Sobieszek, A., in "The Biochemistry of Smooth Muscle" (N. L. Stephens, ed.) p.413, University Park Press, Baltimore, 1977.
3. Walsh, M. P., and Hartshorne, D. J., in "Calcium and Cell Function, Vol. III" (W. Y. Cheung, ed.) p.223, Academic Press, New York, 1982.
4. Adelstein, R. S., Conti, M. A., Hathaway, D. R., and Klee, C. B., J. Biol. Chem. 253:8347 (1978).
5. Conti, M. A., and Adelstein, R. S., J. Biol. Chem. 256:3178 (1981).
6. Dillon, P. F., Aksoy, M. O., Driska, S. P., and Murphy, R. A., Science 211:495 (1981).
7. Chatterjee, M., and Murphy, R. A., Science 221:464 (1983).
8. Siegman, M. J., Butler, T. M., Mooers, S. U., and Davies, R. E., Am. J. Physiol. 231:1501 (1976).

9. Siegman, M. J., Butler, T. M., Mooers, S. U., and Davies, R. E., Science 191:383 (1976).
10. Walters, M., and Marston, S. B., Biochem. J. 197:127 (1981).
11. Chacko, S., and Rosenfeld, A., Proc. Natl. Acad. Sci. USA 78:292 (1982).
12. Nonomura, Y., and Ebashi, S., Biomed. Res. 1:1 (1980).
13. Persechini, A., and Hartshorne, D. J., Science 213:1383 (1981).
14. Ikebe, M., Ogihara, S., and Tonomura, Y., J. Biochem. 91:1809 (1982).
15. Cole, H. A., Patchell, V. B., and Perry, S. V., FEBS Lett. 158:17 (1983).
16. Persechini, A., and Hartshorne, D. J., Biochemistry 22:470 (1983).
17. Sellers, J. R., Chock, P. B., and Adelstein, R. S., Biophys. J. 41:153a (1983).
18. Sellers, J. R., and Adelstein, R. S., Biophys. J. 37:262a (1982).
19. Suzuki, H., Onishi, H., Takahashi, K., and Watanabe, S., J. Biochem. 84:1529 (1978).
20. Suzuki, H., Kamata, T., Onishi, H., and Watanabe, S., J. Biochem. 91:1699 (1982).
21. Onishi, H., and Wakabayashi, T., J. Biochem. 92:871 (1982).
22. Craig, R., Smith, R., and Kendrick-Jones, J., Nature 302:436 (1983).
23. Trybus, K. M., Huiatt, T. W., and Lowey, S., Proc. Natl. Acad. Sci. USA 79:6151 (1982).
24. Ikebe, M., Hinkins, S., and Hartshorne, D. J., Biochemistry 22:4580 (1983).
25. Onishi, H., Suzuki, H., Nakamura, K., Takahashi, K., and Watanabe, S., J. Biochem. 83:835 (1978).
26. Ikebe, M., Hinkins, S., and Hartshorne, D. J., J. Biol. Chem. 258:14770 (1983).
27. Ikebe, M., Tonomura, Y., Onishi, H., and Watanabe, S., J. Biochem. 90:61 (1981).
28. Onishi, H., J. Biochem. 91:157 (1982).
29. Ikebe, M., Onishi, H., and Tonomura Y., J. Biochem. 91:1855 (1982).
30. Gordon, A. R., Proc. Natl. Acad. Sci. USA 75:3527 (1978).
31. Saida, K., and Nonomura, Y., J. Gen. Physiol. 72:1 (1978).
32. Nakahata, N., Pflügers Arch. 382:133 (1979).
33. Nakahata, N., Nakanishi, H., and Suzuki, T., Experientia 37:989 (1981).
34. Arner, A., Pflügers Arch. 397:6 (1983).
35. Somlyo, A. V., Butler, T. M., Bond, M., and Somlyo, A. P., Nature 294:567 (1981).

36. Dabrowska, R., Hinkins, S., Walsh, M. P., and Hartshorne, D. J., Biochem. Biophys. Res. Commun. 107:1524 (1982).
37. Sobue, K., Morimoto, K., Kanda, K., Fukunaga, K., Miyamoto, E., and Kakiuchi, S., Biochem. Int. 5:503 (1982).

Ca REGULATION IN SMOOTH MUSCLE CONTRACTION[1]

Setsuro Ebashi

National Institute for Physiological Sciences
Okazaki

Yoshiaki Nonomura

Department of Pharmacology
Faculty of Medicine
University of Tokyo
Tokyo

Since the present status of the studies on the regulatory mechanisms in smooth muscle was reviewed by Prof. Hartshorne in a previous chapter, this article will describe the views on Ca ion of smooth muscle researchers before the appearance of the present Ca concept and will then refer to particular subjects of smooth muscle regulation on the basis of the leiotonin concept. Emphasis will be laid on the unique nature of smooth muscle quite distinct from skeletal and cardiac muscle (cf. ref. 1).

I. Ca ION IN INTACT SMOOTH MUSCLE

Many muscle scientists had tacitly held the opinion that investigations into skeletal muscle, the muscle with beautiful structure and elegant function, had revealed all the secrets of muscle contraction, and that smooth muscle was nothing but

---

[1]This work was supported in part by Grants-in-Aid for Scientific Research from the Ministry of Education, Science and Culture of Japan, the Muscular Dystrophy Association, and the Iatrochemical Research Foundation.

59

a dull skeletal muscle. Consequently, smooth muscle was rele-
gated to a subordinate position for many years. However, the
finding in 1966(2) that Ca ion was the main carrier of the action current has somewhat changed the situation; it suggested
that smooth muscle itself should be the important subject of
research to clarify the mechanism of muscle contraction.

This reminds us of the epoch-making discovery of Ringer in
1883 (3) using frog heart, which implied the essential role of
Ca ion in contractile processes. This finding, however, was
somewhat distorted by another important finding made by him-
self in 1886 (4) that the removal of Ca ion from the bathing
medium induced repetitive twitches of skeletal muscle. To
reconcile these apparently contradictory findings, the ratio
between Ca and K ions was stressed as the key factor main-
taining the physiological states of muscle, i.e., a rhyth-
mically contracting state for cardiac muscle and a quiescent
state, unless stimulated, for skeletal muscle, thus
distracting scientific attention from the direct action of Ca
ion on the contractile system.

A question then may arise why smooth muscle, of which the
action current is completely Ca dependent, could not play a
substantial role in the development of the Ca concept.
Indeed, experiments similar to those conducted by Ringer with
frog heart were reported early in this century using various
kinds of smooth muscle (5,6). However, all of them were
carried out under the influence of Ringer's work, so their
results were all interpreted on the basis of Ca/K ratio.[1]

---

[1]There are some indications that smooth muscle contraction
can take place without Ca ion; for instance, catecholamine
induced the contraction of intact vas deferens which had been
subjected to exhaustive washing with EGTA for several days
(7). Two cases of muscle contraction without Ca ion are well
known (several chemical agents of completely nonphysiological
nature can also produce the contraction of muscle fiber
models). One is that low concentrations of ATP can induce the
contraction of skeletal muscle contractile systems in the
complete absence of Ca ion; this is the fundamental property
of skeletal muscle actomyosin (see Fig. 2). The other is that
high concentrations of free Mg ion, 4 mM or more, bring about
slow but steady tension development of smooth muscle skinned
fibers without Ca ion (8). The latter phenomenon has not been
well explained, but it must somehow be related to known findings, e.g., the Mg effect on myosin filament formation or Mg-
dependence of the function of smooth muscle actin. Compared
with these, the mechanism of the contraction of smooth muscle
mentioned is beyond our present knowledge; however, this cannot play a part in physiological contractile processes.

In this way, the direct role of Ca ion in contractility was never proposed in heart and smooth muscle research. Soon after the conclusive demonstration of the role of Ca in the contractile system of skeletal muscle (9, cf. 10), there appeared a few papers that explained the action of Ca ion in smooth muscle based on today's concept (11,12). It was interesting but puzzling that the Ca concept was first established in skeletal muscle, where Ca ion in the outer medium has nothing to do with the contractile processes.

II. Ca ION IN SMOOTH MUSCLE CONTRACTILE SYSTEM

In spite of the pioneering work of Ringer, the role of Ca ion in the actomyosin-ATP system of cardiac muscle was not confirmed until 1964, several years after establishment of the Ca concept in skeletal muscle.

This was also true of smooth muscle. In 1965, Bohr's group presented a landmark paper (13) confirming the activating effect of Ca ion, using glycerinated muscle fibers (Figs. 1 and 2). This paper revealed many important properties of smooth muscle, for instance, the necessity of a sig-

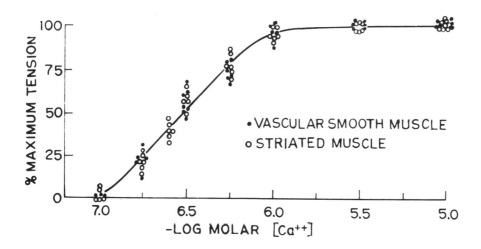

FIGURE 1. Ca ion concentrations and tension developed by the glycerinated fibers of skeletal (psoas) and smooth (vascular) muscle (cited from Filo et al. (13)). Conditions: temperature 20°C; 150 mM KCl; 20 mM histidine buffer (pH 6.6); 5 mM ATP and 5 mM Mg; 4 mM EGTA; appropriate concentrations of Ca.

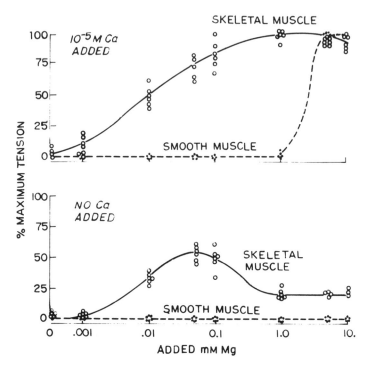

FIGURE 2. Effect of Mg ion on tension development (cited from Filo et al. (13)). Conditions: essentially the same as those in the legend to Fig. 1 except that no Mg was included in the standard solution and 0.5 mM EGTA was used to produce Ca ion concentrations of 10^{-5} M and zero. Tension development of smooth muscle started at 1×10^{-3} M and reached maximum at about 5×10^{-3} M added Mg. Since 5 mM ATP exists in the medium, the free Mg ion concentrations under these conditions are about 4×10^{-5} M and 9×10^{-4} M, respectively, the latter being close to the physiological concentration of Mg ion in the cytoplasm. In an in vitro system, 4-5 mM Mg ion is necessary for filament formation of myosin as well as for contractile response of the smooth muscle actomyosin system. This discrepancy may be largely explained by the difference in myosin concentration.

nificant amount of free Mg ion for contractility, which is now interpreted as being indispensable for the filament formation of myosin (14).

Demonstration of the Ca effect on ATPase activity as well as on the superprecipitation of extracted contractile proteins was also done in the same year (15) using chicken gizzard muscle.

III. CHARACTERISTIC FEATURES OF SMOOTH MUSCLE CONTRACTILE PROTEINS

As has been emphasized, the most important characteristics of smooth muscle is the quiescent state of pure actomyosin in the presence of ATP. In other words, actin and myosin do not positively react with each other in the presence of ATP, a factor(s) being necessary for activation together with Ca ion (16). Thus Ca ion acts as a true activator in smooth muscle in contrast with the case in skeletal muscle where Ca ion acts as a de-repressor, removing the suppression induced by troponin in the absence of Ca ion.

Another important feature of the smooth muscle actomyosin system is the monophasic type of response to the increase in MgATP concentrations, i.e., no clear biphasic type response or 'substrate-inhibition' type response is exhibited (Fig. 3), in sharp contrast with the skeletal muscle actomyosin system (16).

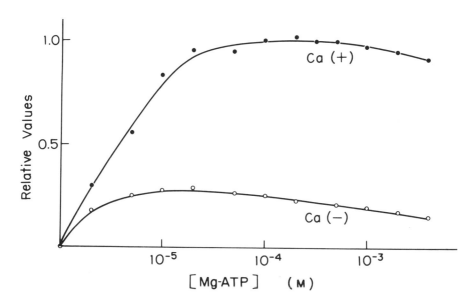

FIGURE 3. Relationship between MgATP concentration and superprecipitation of gizzard myosin B (cited from ref. 16). Relative absorbancies 20 min after addition of ATP were plotted against MgATP concentration. In the absence of Ca ion, the relationship becomes slightly biphasic, though it is not comparable with that of the skeletal muscle contractile system shown in Fig. 2 (lower).

Generally speaking, smooth muscle actomyosin is less sensitive to the change in ionic strength than the skeletal one, but this difference is not so marked as the above (16)[1].

In addition to the effect of Mg ion on myosin mentioned earlier, smooth muscle actin is also dependent on Mg ion in its reaction with myosin in the presence of ATP (17).

Smooth muscle tropomyosin is also distinct from the skeletal one. Under ordinary conditions, it does not replace the latter in the troponin system, but this is due to its strong activating effect of the actin–myosin–ATP interaction, the effect which is not found in skeletal tropomyosin. However, smooth muscle tropomyosin can cooperate with troponin under special conditions, where its activating effect is counteracted by some means, e.g., using relatively high ionic strength or high ATP concentration.

The failure of skeletal tropomyosin in replacing smooth muscle tropomyosin in smooth muscle regulation can be attributed to its lack of the activating effect mentioned above. However, this does not mean that the activating effect is the main function of tropomyosin in the smooth muscle regulation, because if we use special experimental conditions, skeletal tropomyosin can somehow be utilized by the smooth muscle regulatory system.

IV. THE FACTS NOT CONSISTENT WITH THE MYSOSIN LIGHT CHAIN KINASE THEORY

The majority of research workers on smooth muscle are of the opinion that Ca dependent myosin light chain kinase is the physiological activator of the smooth muscle actomyosin system (cf. the chapter by Prof. Hartshorne). We were able to con-

---

[1]Protein concentration, particularly the local concentration in the actomyosin gel, is an important factor in the sensitivity of the contractile system to the ionic strength. Fiber models, such as glycerinated fibers or skinned fibers that have a high local concentration of actomyosin, and reconstituted actomyosin which is strongly hydrated are two extremes, the least and most sensitive systems, respectively (acto-HMM-S1 is far more sensitive than reconstituted actomyosin, but this may not be considered on the same level as the above). However, even if we use the same protein concentration, natural actomyosin is less sensitive than reconstituted actomyosin. The reason for this is not yet known.

firm the results obtained by the group favoring the kinase concept. For instance, the assertion of Chacko et al. (19) that stably phosphorylated myosin vigorously reacts with actin in the presence of ATP, irrespective of the presence or absence of Ca ion, was confirmed by using pure myosin (S. Nakamura, personal communication).

However, there are several pieces of evidence which cannot be explained by the kinase theory. As shown in Fig. 4, if actin is added to myosin immediately after its phosphorylation, no marked activation is noticed in the absence of Ca ion, in spite of retention of the phosphorylated

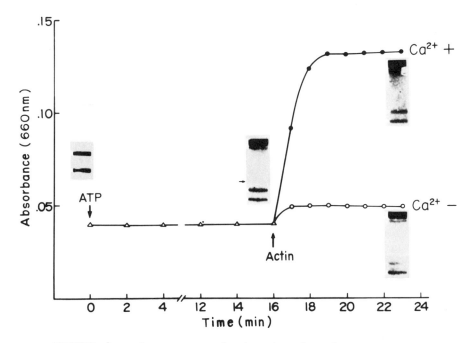

FIGURE 4. Responses of phosphorylated myosin to actin. Gizzard myosin was incubated with crude light chain kinase free of phosphatase, tropomyosin and calmodulin in medium containing 0.02 M KCl, 8 mM $MgCl_2$, 0.02 M Tris-maleate buffer (pH 6.8) and 0.1 mM $CaCl_2$ (without using Ca-EGTA buffer) and at a certain point gizzard actin in a small volume, one thirtieth the total volume, was added: one was actin only and the other actin together with EGTA to a final concentration of 1 mM (for further details, see ref. 20). Note that virtually no dephosphorylation took place in the absence of Ca ion (if we look carefully, a slight dephosphorylation, about 10%, took place in the final stage), and that little activation was seen in spite of nearly full phosphorylation.

state of myosin[1] (20).

Another important observation is that some crude leiotonin preparations containing kinase but not calmodulin, can activate the actin-myosin interaction in the absence of calmodulin without phosphorylating light chain (21) (Fig. 5).

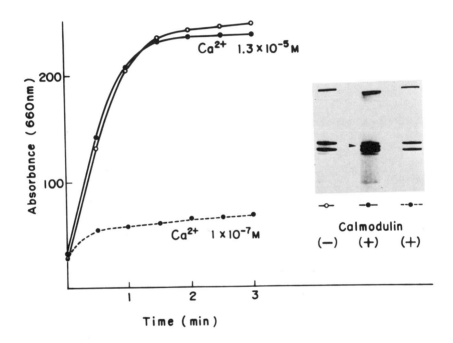

FIGURE 5.   Superprecipitation without phosphorylation. Crude leiotonin preparation treated with Ultrogel (AC44) activated the actomyosin without calmodulin (o) to almost the same extent as that with calmodulin (•). Nearly full phosphorylation took place in the latter, whereas no phosphorylation was seen in the former (for details see Fig. 3 of ref. 21).

---

[1]Recently it has been shown that in the case of myosin from which phosphatase has been completely removed by special procedures, phosphorylation always produces an immediate contractile response irrespective of the presence or absence of Ca ion (S. Nakamura, personal communication). The myosin preparation used in the above experiment contained a small amount of phosphatase, but in an amount so small that it showed virtually no dephosphorylation even in the absence of Ca ion as indicated above. The difference between these two results, therefore, cannot be ascribed simply to the presence or absence of phosphatase.

The discrepancy between the activation of the actomyosin system and myosin light chain phosphorylation can be seen in ammonium sulfate fractions. As shown in Fig. 6, the fractions soluble and insoluble in high ammonium sulfate concentrations respectively contain high and low kinase activities compared with the activating effect (21). Sometimes we can obtain the fraction which exhibits strong activation effect but virtually no kinase activity. Such a fraction is more easily obtained from aged and/or once frozen preparations; the reason for this is not yet understood.

Skeletal muscle light chain kinase is much less effective on gizzard myosin, but if used in a large amount, it exerts the same degree of phosphorylating activity as does gizzard kinase. Under this condition its activating effect on the gizzard actomyosin system is much weaker than the kinase derived from the gizzard.

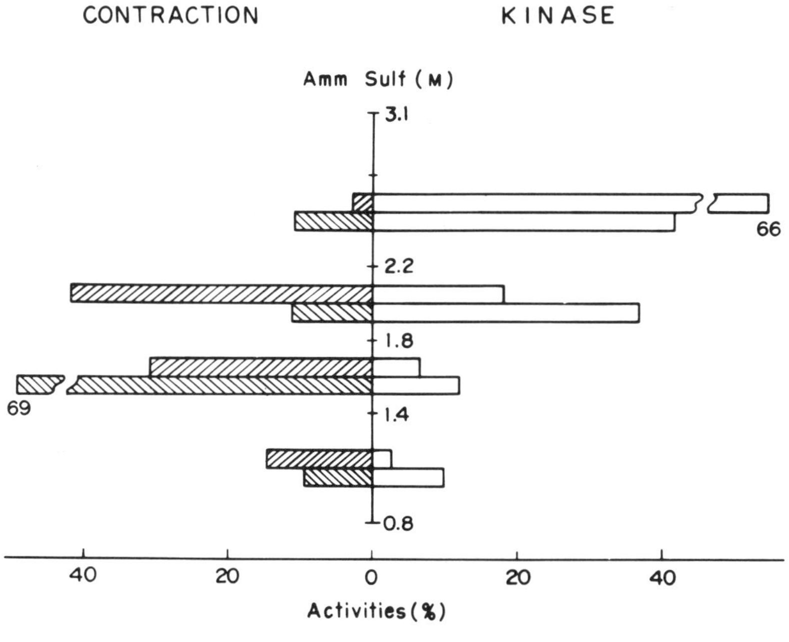

FIGURE 6. Actomyosin-activating and myosin-phosphorylating effects of fractions obtained by inverse ammonium sulfate fractionation. Two cases are illustrated. Bar lengths indicate the activities in relative values (total, 100) of the fractions precipitated at ammonium sulfate concentrations between the values shown above and below the bars (for inverse ammonium sulfate fractionation and other details see ref. 18).

All these findings strongly indicate that even if myosin light chain phosphorylation is an important activation mechanism, it cannot explain the whole events concerned with the smooth muscle activation.

V. SEARCH FOR LEIOTONIN

Since the leiotonin concept has been reviewed elsewhere (1,22), the description here will be confined to results that are at variance with those stated previously.

We once reported on purified leiotonin (leiotonin A) of a molecular weight around 80,000 daltons (23). Increasing our efforts to avoid protein degradation by various procedures including the use of protease inhibitors, it became very difficult to reproduce those earlier results. Recently, we were able to prepare almost the same preparation as previously reported under certain conditions, and in this case we noticed a slight but significant protein degradation. Therefore, it is likely that the previous leiotonin A preparation was apparently a proteolytic product of native leiotonin A.

The effort to isolate the original leiotonin in a homogeneous state is continuing. Preliminary results indicate that the protein resembles myosin light chain kinase in many respects except for its kinase activity. At present we do not know how to interpret this puzzling result.

VI. SUMMARY

The change of views on the role of Ca ion in smooth muscle contraction has been historically reviewed. Emphasis has been given to the fact that traditional or conventional concepts had prevented smooth muscle scientists from recognizing the importance of Ca ion as the direct activator of the contractile system in smooth muscle.

This was followed by the presentation of results which are inconsistent with the idea that myosin phosphorylation should be the essential step, perhaps the sole one, in activating the contractile processes of smooth muscle. Brief reference was also made to the recent results of studies on the leiotonin system.

REFERENCES

1. Ebashi, S., Proc. Roy. Soc. Lond. B 207:259 (1980).
2. Nonomura, Y., Hotta, Y., and Ohashi, H., Science 152:97 (1966).
3. Ringer, S., J. Physiol. 4:29 (1883).
4. Ringer, S., J. Physiol. 7:291 (1886).
5. Stiles, P. G., Am. J. Physiol. 5:338 (1901).
6. Evans, C. L., Physiol. Rev. 6:358 (1926).
7. Ashoori, F., and Tomita, T., J. Physiol. 338:165 (1983).
8. Saida, K., and Nonomura, Y., J. Gen. Physiol. 72:1 (1978).
9. Ebashi, S., J. Biochem. 48:150 (1960).
10. Ebashi, S., and Endo, M., Progr. Biophys. 18:123 (1968).
11. Yukisada, N., Folia Pharmacol. Japon. 56:936 (1960); Yukisada, N., and Ebashi, F., Jap. J. Pharmacol. 11:46 (1961).
12. Edman, K. A. P., and Schild, H. O., Nature 190:350 (1961); J. Physiol. 161:424 (1962).
13. Filo, R. S., Bohr, D. F., and Ruegg, J. C., Science 147:1581 (1965).
14. Nonomura, Y., in "Cell Motility: Molecules and Organization" (S. Hatano et al., eds.), p. 467. University of Tokyo Press, Tokyo, 1979.
15. Iwakura, H., Tokyo J. Med. Sci. 75:49 (1965).
16. Ebashi, S., Nonomura, Y., Toyo-oka, T., and Katayama, E., in Calcium in Biological System. Symp. Soc. Exp. Biol. 30:349 (1976).
17. Mikawa, T., and Maruyama, K., Proc. Jap. Acad. B 57:23 (1981).
18. Ebashi, S., Mikawa, T., Hirata, M., and Nonomura, Y., Ann. N. Y. Acad. Sci. 307:451 (1978).
19. Chacko, S., Conti, M. A., and Adelstein, R. S., Proc. Natl. Acad. Sci. USA 74:129 (1977).
20. Ebashi, S., Nakamura, S., Nakasone, H., Kohama, K., and Nonomura, Y., in "Calcium Modulators" (T. Godfraind et al., eds.), p. 39. Elsevier Biomedical Press, Amsterdam, 1982.
21. Ebashi, S., and Nakasone, H., Proc. Jap. Acad. B 57:217 (1981).
22. Nonomura, Y., and Ebashi, S., Biomed. Res., 1:1 (1980).
23. Mikawa, T., Toyo-oka, T., Nonomura, Y., and Ebashi, S., J. Biochem. 81:273 (1977).

EFFECTS OF Ca^{2+} AND Mg^{2+} ON ACTIN POLYMERIZATION

Thomas D. Pollard

Department of Cell Biology and Anatomy
Johns Hopkins Medical School
Baltimore, Maryland

I. INTRODUCTION

Actin is the central element of the contractile apparatus in muscle and in non-muscle cells. Consequently, it is important to understand in detail how the actin molecule assembles into actin filaments. Although it has been known for over 25 years that the polymerization mechanism includes a slow nucleation step followed by a rapid elongation step (reviewed by Oosawa and Kasai, ref. 1), it is remarkable that relatively little has been learned about the quantitative aspects of the polymerization process. It was not until 1981 that the absolute value of any of the rate constants in the polymerization process was measured (2).

In this paper I will review briefly the work that we have done to identify the steps in the actin polymerization process, to evaluate the rate constants for these steps and to learn how the divalent cations Ca^{2+} and Mg^{2+} affect these reactions. Much of this work has been carried out by my colleague, Dr. John A. Cooper (3).

II. METHODS FOR THE ANALYSIS OF THE FULL POLYMERIZATION MECHANISM

Table I presents a simple model for actin polymerization that consists of 4 separate reversible steps. Similar models have been studied by Tobacman and Korn (4) and Frieden (5). The first step is a first order reaction during which individual actin monomers are activated in some way that promotes

TABLE   I. Kinetic Constants for Actin Polymerization

Steps in Actin Polymerization in KCl plus		Mg^{2+} or Ca^{2+}	
Activation	$A_1 \underset{k_2}{\overset{k_1}{\rightleftharpoons}} A_1^*$	k_1 (s^{-1}) 0.05	---
		k_2 (s^{-1}) $[k_1/100]$	
Nucleation	$nA_1 \underset{k_4}{\overset{k_3}{\rightleftharpoons}} A_n$	n 3	3
		k_3 $(M^{-1}s^{-1})$ 6000	400
		k_4 (s^{-1}) $[500]$	
Elongation	$A_1 + A_i \underset{k_6}{\overset{k_5}{\rightleftharpoons}} A_{i+1}$	k_5 $(M^{-1}s^{-1})$ $\sim10^7$	$\sim10^7$
		k_6 (s^{-1}) 2	6
Fragmentation	$A_i \overset{k_7}{\longrightarrow} A_j + A_k$	k_7 (s^{-1}) ---	10^{-14}

Mechanism and data from Cooper et al. (3). Values in brackets
were defined, not measured.   --- means that this reaction was
not   required   to   fit   the   computed   kinetic   curves   to   the
experimental data.

their ability to form actin filaments. The second step is
nucleation. The three important parameters for this step are
the number of actin monomers in the nucleus, n, and the association and dissociation rate constants. The third step is
the elongation reaction. Here, an actin filament consisting
of i subunits binds an actin monomer to increase its length by
1. This is a reversible reaction characterized by a second
order association rate constant and a first order dissociation
rate constant. The final step is referred to as fragmentation. Here an actin filament breaks into 2 shorter filaments. The reverse reaction, called annealing, is the end to
end association of 2 actin filaments to form one longer actin
filament. We have not considered annealing in our analysis.
    Of the 4 separate steps postulated in this mechanism, only
the third step, elongation, can be evaluated directly at the
present time. Consequently, indirect assays are required to

identify which of these steps occur during the actin self-assembly process and to evalute the rate constants for the steps. The published data (3) was obtained with rabbit skeletal muscle actin, but we have obtained essentially identical results with Acanthamoeba actin.

Our analysis began with measuring the absolute value of the elongation rate constants directly by electron microscopy (Table I). More details on the subtle effects of divalent cations on elongation reactions are considered below. Then we used fluorometry to measure the time course of pyrene-labeled actin polymerization as a function of the actin monomer concentration. These data were used to detect and analyze the other steps in the process.

Activation: Using a plot of the log of the inverse delay time at the outset of polymerization vs. the log of the actin concentration, we are able to establish whether a first order rate limiting activation step is present under a given set of conditions. For example, if the slope of the log-log plot is close to 1.0 then a first order activation step is necessary in the reaction mechanism. If the slope of such a log-log plot is higher than 1.5, activation may occur but it is not necessary to include an activation step in the reaction mechanism.

Evaluation of nucleus size and rate constants: We used a computer to select the nucleus size and the single set of activation, nucleation and fragmentation rate constants that best fit the dependence of the polymerization time course on the actin concentration. To simplify the calculations we assumed a steady-state nucleation mechanism with a single association rate constant as suggested and justified by Wegner and Engel (6). We arbitrarily assigned the nucleation dissociation rate constant, k_4, a value of 500 per second. The consequence of these assumptions is that we determine the ratio of k_3 to k_4 rather than the absolute value of the association rate constant for nucleation.

Even though the reaction mechanism (Table I) is simple, it is able to account quantitatively for the time course of actin polymerization over at least a 6 fold range of actin monomer concentrations. The fit between the theoretical curves calculated with the rate constants selected by the computer is remarkably close to the experimental data. This gives us confidence that we have identified correctly the steps in the polymerization mechanism and that we have been able to identify at least the correct order of magnitude for the rate constants at each step.

III. THE MECHANISM OF ACTIN POLYMERIZATION IN Ca^{2+} OR Mg^{2+}

The results summarized in Table I explain why actin poly-
merizes so much more rapidly in Mg^{2+} than in Ca^{2+}. The most
important factor is that actin forms nuclei at much higher
rates in Mg^{2+} than Ca^{2+}. In Mg^{2+} the ratio of the association
rate constant for nucleation, k_3, to the dissociation rate
constant, k_4, is at least an order of magnitude larger than it
is in Ca^{2+}. Either the association rate constant is larger or
the dissociation rate constant is smaller in Mg^{2+} than in
Ca^{2+}. Tobacman and Korn (4) used similar techniques to show
that nucleation is faster in Mg^{2+} than in Ca^{2+}. Under the
conditions used in Table I, the elongation is also faster in
Mg^{2+} than in Ca^{2+}, because the dissociation rate constant is
smaller in Mg^{2+}. However, these differences make a relatively
minor contribution to the differences in the overall time
course of polymerization.

The activation step is rate limiting and is probably present in only Mg^{2+}. This suggested to us that the activation
reaction might in fact be the exchange of Ca^{2+} bound to the
high affinity site on actin for Mg^{2+} in the buffer. A similar
conclusion has been reached subsequently by Freiden (5). The
activation step has about the same first order rate constant
as the exchange of Mg^{2+} for Ca^{2+} bound to actin that Freiden
has measured by an independent method (7).

Another difference between polymerization in Mg^{2+} and
Ca^{2+} is the necessity to include a fragmentation step in the
mechanism in Ca^{2+}. It is possible that the Mg^{2+} filaments may
be more stable than the Ca^{2+} actin filaments, but it is also
possible that this very slow step only becomes apparent when
the polymerization process is exceedingly slow as in the presence of Ca^{2+}. It may be that polymerization is too fast in
the presence of Mg^{2+} for this step to be detected.

In addition to the profound effects that Ca^{2+} and Mg^{2+}
have on the nucleation rate, they also have interesting, but
somewhat subtle, effects on the elongation reaction. Figure 1
and Fig. 2 show experiments carried out with a fluorometric
assay for the actin polymer concentration. They are plots of
the rate of elongation from preformed actin filament nuclei as
a function of the actin monomer concentration. The slopes of
these plots are proportional to the elongation association
rate constant and the Y-intercepts are proportional to the
dissociation rate constants. The X-intercept is the critical
concentration. All of these experiments were carried out in
the presence of 50 mM KCl, 0.1 mM $CaCl_2$ and 0.1 mM ATP.
Without any additions to this reaction mixture, the elongation
rate is low and the critical concentration is high, about 3.5
μM. The slope of the plots is higher if either EGTA is added

to chelate the Ca^{2+} or if millimolar concentrations of Mg^{2+} are included. Considering first the effect of the Mg^{2+}, note that the dissociation rate constant becomes much smaller and that the association rate constant (the slope) is 4 times higher in 2 mM Mg^{2+} than in the absence of Mg^{2+}. At intermediate concentrations of Mg^{2+} there is a gradual increase in the association rate constant as shown in the inset. In the presence of EGTA both the association and dissociation rate

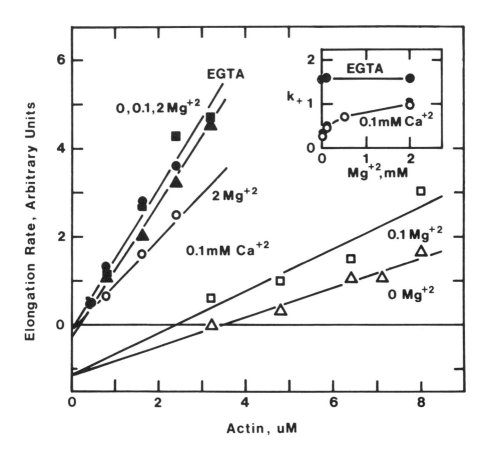

FIGURE 1. Dependence of the elongation rate on the concentration of <u>Acanthamoeba</u> actin monomer. Conditions: 50 mM KCl, 10 mM imidazole (pH 7), 0.1 mM $CaCl_2$, 0.1 mM ATP, 0.5 μM actin filaments as nuclei. Some samples (closed symbols) had 1 mM EGTA. The concentration of $MgCl_2$ was varied. The inset shows how the slope of these plots (k_+) depends on the Mg^{2+} concentration. In calculating k_+ (arbitrary units) it was assumed that the nucleus concentration was the same for all conditions.

constants become independent of the concentration of Mg^{2+} in
the range of 0 to 2 mM. One interpretation (Fig. 3) of these
data is that Ca^{2+} bound to low affinity sites on the actin
molecule (8) influences the elongation rate constants. When
Ca^{2+} is bound to these low affinity sites the association rate
constant is low and the dissociation rate constant is high.
This loosely bound Ca^{2+} can be displaced from the actin mole-

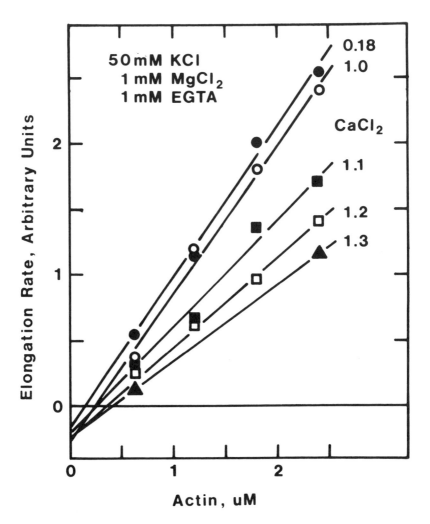

FIGURE 2. Dependence of the elongation rate on the concentration of <u>Acathamoeba</u> actin monomer. Conditions: 50 mM
KCl, 10 mM imidazole (pH 7), 1.0 mM $MgCl_2$, 1.0 mM EGTA, 0.1 mM
ATP. The total Ca (given to the right of each curve in millimolar) was varied by adding $CaCl_2$.

cules either by millimolar concentrations of Mg^{2+} or simply by the inclusion of EGTA in the reaction mixture. Since both EGTA and Mg^{2+} exert their effect by removing loosely bound Ca^{2+}, the combination of EGTA and Mg^{2+} gives results similar to either one of these agents alone. The tightly bound divalent cation may have lesser effects on the elongation process, because both low and high elongation rates can be attained with Ca^{2+} bound to the high affinity site. I have not carried out experiments under conditions where Mg^{2+} is bound to the high affinity site and Ca^{2+} is bound to the low affinity sites.

The hypothesis that Ca^{2+} on the low affinity sites modulates the elongation rate is supported by the experiments shown in Fig. 2. Here again the elongation rate is plotted as a function of the actin concentration. The reactions are carried in 50 mM KCl with 1 mM $MgCl_2$, 1 mM EGTA and 0.1 mM ATP. The free Ca^{2+} is varied by the addition of $CaCl_2$. The total Ca concentration in these samples was measured by atomic absorption spectrophotometry. When the total Ca^{2+} concentration exceeds the EGTA concentration there is a progressive concentration dependent inhibition of the association rate constant. Over the range of 0 to 0.3 mM free Ca^{2+}, one would expect Ca^{2+} to displace the Mg^{2+} from the low affinity sites on the actin molecule, because the affinity for Ca^{2+} at these sites is approximately 25 times higher than the affinity for Mg^{2+} (7).

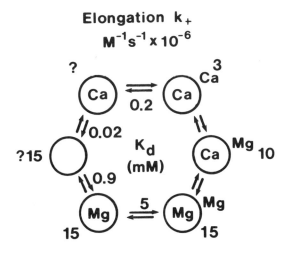

Elongation k_+

$M^{-1}s^{-1} \times 10^{-6}$

FIGURE 3. Comparison of estimates of the elongation association rate constant (k_+) and the dissociation constants for binding of Ca^{2+} and Mg^{2+} to actin. The dissociation constants are from Strzelecka-Golaszewska et al. (8) and Frieden (7).

A tentative interpretation of the effect of divalent cations on actin filament elongation are shown in Fig. 3. Here the tightly bound divalent cation is pictured inside the actin molecule and the loosely bound divalent cation is shown on the surface. Around the inside of this scheme note the dissociation constants for the divalent cations that have been estimated by Strzelecka-Golaszewska et al. (8) and Frieden (7). There are actually multiple low affinity sites (8).

Around the periphery of the diagram note my estimates of the elongation association rate constant for these different species. This model suggests that actin monomers having no loosely bound divalent cations or Mg^{2+} bound to these low affinity sites have a high association rate constant. The absolute value of this rate constants, $10-20 \times 10^6$ M^{-1} s^{-1}, is in the range where the reaction rate may be limited by diffusion. In contrast, actin monomers with Ca^{2+} bound to the low affinity site probably have a much smaller association rate constant. It is possible that the binding of the actin monomer to the end of the filament is limited by these Ca^{2+} ions. The concentrations of free Mg^{2+} and Ca^{2+} in the cell probably mean that these low affinity sites are rarely occupied by Ca^{2+}, but this remains a potential mechanism for modulating actin assembly in the cell.

IV. ACTIN-BINDING PROTEINS FROM ACANTHAMOEBA

In the cell the polymerization of the actin is controlled by a variety of accessory protein molecules that intervene in this polymerization process at one or more steps in the reaction mechanism. In the Acanthamoeba three different classes of actin regulatory proteins have been identified (Table II).

The first class is represented by the small soluble protein called profilin. Profilin binds to actin monomers and regulates polymerization by limiting the concentration of free actin (9,10,11,12). Under physiological conditions (50 mM KCl, 1 mM $MgCl_2$, 1 mM EGTA) profilin strongly inhibits the nucleation steps of the assembly mechanism. Assuming that profilin acts at this step simply by altering the concentration of free actin monomers and that only free actin monomers can participate in nucleation, we estimate using the same curve fitting approach that we employed for estimating the nucleation and activation rate constants that the dissociation constant for the actin profilin complex is 5 μM. In contrast, under the same conditions profilin inhibits the elongation step only very weakly. If this effect of profilin were due simply to the formation of an actin-profilin complex that could not participate in elongation, then the dissociation

Table II. <u>Acanthamoeba</u> Actin-binding Proteins

Class	Subunit Composition	Ref.
Monomer Binding Protein		
Profilin	12,000	9,10,11,12
Filament Capping Proteins		
Capping protein	29,000 + 31,000	13
Filament Crosslinking Proteins		
Gelactin-I	23,000	16
Gelactin-II	28,000	16
Gelactin-III	33,000	16
Gelactin-IV	38,000	16
Gelation protein	2 x 90,000	18
Spectrin	? 2 x 250,000	20

constant for the actin profilin complex would be approximately 100 μM. Our explanation for the difference in these apparent dissociation constants is that the actin-profilin complex can bind the end of an actin filament. Once the complex binds, the affinity of profilin for actin is markedly lower than its affinity for the free actin monomer. This leads to rapid dissociation of profilin from the end of the actin filament and accounts for the apparent low affinity of profilin on the elongation reaction. This is equivalent to saying that profilin binds to the end(s) of actin filaments with a dissociation constant of 100 μM. The presence or absence of Ca^{2+} has no substantial effect on the affinity of profilin for actin. This suggests that Ca^{2+} does not regulate the association of actin and profilin unless a third protein is involved.

The second class of actin regulatory proteins affects polymerization by binding to one end of the actin filament. The first protein in this category was named capping protein (13). It binds to the barbed end of actin filaments and prevents the addition of actin subunits at that end. The <u>Acanthamoeba</u> capping protein also influences the nucleation reaction. It stimulates the formation of nuclei by stabilizing actin dimers which then go on to form nuclei. As in the case of profilin the effect of the capping protein on actin polymerization is not regulated by Ca^{2+}. There are a number of examples of capping proteins in other cells, such as villin (14) and gelsolin (15) that are regulated by Ca^{2+}, so we expect eventually to find such Ca^{2+} regulated capping proteins in the Acanthamoeba as well.

The third type of actin regulatory protein crosslinks actin filaments into networks and bundles. The Acanthamoeba has four actin crosslinking proteins that have been called gelactins (16). They are not regulated by Ca^{2+} (17). Acanthamoeba also has a protein similar to alpha-actinin that we call gelation protein (18). The gelation protein consists of two 90,000 MW polypeptide chains. It is a rod-shaped molecule 50 nm long and about 3 nm wide. It binds only weakly to actin filaments (the dissociation constant is larger than 5 μM), but even at low concentrations it effectively crosslinks actin filaments into continuous 3-dimensional networks. This is possible because the actin filaments are so long. The initial experiments showed that polymerization of actin in the presence of gelation protein and $MgCl_2$ gave a higher apparent viscosity at low shear rates if EGTA was present rather than Ca^{2+}. This led to the conclusion (18) that the gelation protein might be regulated by Ca^{2+}. However, more detailed studies (19) have revealed that the effect of Ca^{2+} is on the actin, not on the gelation protein. As described above actin assembles more rapidly in EGTA than in Ca^{2+} even with Mg^{2+} present, so samples with EGTA had higher viscosities simply due to the fact that the actin polymer concentration was higher at early time points that were assayed.

At this point 8 different actin binding proteins have been purified from the Acanthamoeba. It is remarkable that none of these proteins seems to be regulated by the Ca^{2+} ion concentration. If Ca^{2+} controls the actin assembly in Acanthamoeba it may do so by acting directly on the actin. However, it seems more likely that the cell has Ca^{2+} sensitive actin-binding proteins that have not yet been identified or that calmodulin or other Ca^{2+}-binding modulator proteins confer Ca^{2+}-sensitivity on one or more of the proteins already under investigation.

REFERENCES

1. Oosawa, F. and Kasai, M., in "Subunits in Biological
    Systems, Part A" (S. N. Timasheff, and G. D. Fasman,
    eds.), p. 261. Marsel Dekker, New York, 1971.
2. Pollard, T. D., and Mooseker, M. S., J. Cell Biol. 88:654
    (1981).
3. Cooper, J. A., Buhle, E. L., Jr., Walker, S. B., Tsong,
    T. Y., and Pollard, T. D., Biochemistry 22:2193 (1983).
4. Tobacman, L., and Korn, E. D., J. Biol. Chem. 258:3207
    (1983).
5. Frieden, C., Proc. Natl. Acad. Sci. USA 80:6513 (1983).
6. Wegner, A., and Engel, J., Biophys. Chem. 3:215 (1975).
7. Frieden, C., J. Biol. Chem. 257:2882 (1982).
8. Strzelecka-Golaszewska, H., Prochniewicz, E., and
    Drabikowski, W., Eur. J. Biochem. 88:229 (1978).
9. Tobacman, L. S., and Korn, E. D., J. Biol. Chem. 257:4166
    (1982).
10. Tseng, P., and Pollard, T. D., J. Cell Biol. 94:213
    (1982).
11. Tobacman, L. S., Brenner, S. L., and Korn, E. D., J.
    Biol. Chem. 258:8806 (1983).
12. Pollard, T. D., and Cooper, J. A., (Submitted).
13. Isenberg, G. H., Aebi, U., and Pollard, T. D., Nature
    288:455 (1980).
14. Glenney, J. R., Kaulfus, P., and Weber, K., Cell 24:471
    (1981).
15. Yin, H. L., Zaner, K. S., and Stossel, T. P., J. Biol.
    Chem. 255:9494 (1980).
16. Maruta, H., and Korn, E. D., J. Biol. Chem. 252:399
    (1977).
17. MacLean-Fletcher, S., and Pollard, T. D., J. Cell Biol.
    85:414 (1980).
18. Pollard, T. D., J. Biol. Chem. 256:7666 (1981).
19. Bichell, D., Rimm, D., and Pollard, T. D., (in Prepa-
    ration).
20. Pollard, T. D., Cell Motility, 3:693 (1983).

PART II.
CALCIUM CHANNEL AND TRANSMEMBRANE CONTROL

PHOSPHODIESTERASE-CATALYSED BREAKDOWN OF PHOSPHATIDYLINOSITOL 4,5-BISPHOSPHATE INITIATES RECEPTOR-STIMULATED INOSITOL LIPID METABOLISM[1]

Robert H. Michell
Phillip T. Hawkins
Sue Palmer
Christopher J. Kirk

Department of Biochemistry
University of Birmingham
Birmingham, U.K.

I. INTRODUCTION

The stimulation of many cell-surface receptors evokes an increase in the turnover of inositol lipids. Activation of many or all of these receptors also: (a) raises cytosol Ca^{2+} concentration, (b) activates protein kinase C, (c) elevates the cellular cyclic GMP concentration, and (d) mobilizes arachidonate as a precursor of prostaglandins, leukotrienes and other pharmacologically active agents. For some years, it has seemed possible that receptor-stimulated breakdown of an inositol lipid might be the single receptor-coupled biochemical reaction responsible for initiating all of these diverse signalling events (for reviews, see refs. 1-8).

If stimulated inositol lipid metabolism is indeed essential for this cellular information flow, then it is essential that we should understand the initial event that triggers these widespread and striking changes. Between 1973 and 1980, our laboratory played a major role in establishing that cellular depletion of phosphatidylinositol (PtdIns) is a feature

[1]This work has been supported by project grants and research studentships from the Medical Research Council of the U.K.

CALCIUM REGULATION
IN BIOLOGICAL SYSTEMS

common to all situations in which receptors activate inositol lipid metabolism. As a result, there has been widespread acceptance of the view that receptors somehow control the activation of a phosphodiesterase that degrades PtdIns, yielding 1,2-diacylglycerol and a mixture of inositol 1-phosphate and inositol 1,2-cyclic phosphate. Early in this work, we realised that the water-soluble product(s) released inside cells as a result of inositol lipid degradation would be prime candidates as intracellular messengers. We therefore suggested that inositol 1,2-cyclic phosphate might have such a second messenger role (9), but no convincing evidence of its ability to control any cell function was ever forthcoming (1).

It now appears that this emphasis on the importance of PtdIns hydrolysis was misplaced. Work in a large number of laboratories since 1980 has demonstrated that the lipid whose breakdown is controlled by receptors is phosphatidylinositol 4,5-bisphosphate (PtdIns4,5P_2) rather than PtdIns, and that the 'PtdIns breakdown' recorded in earlier experiments represented the depletion of PtdIns that was caused by its utilisation for resynthesis of PtdIns4,5P_2 concentration, in the face of the receptor-stimulated breakdown of this lipid. Thus the products of this putative information-transducing reaction are now seen to be 1,2-diacylglycerol (as with PtdIns hydrolysis) and inositol 1,4,5-trisphosphate (rather than inositol 1-phosphate and inositol 1,2-cyclic phosphate). Studies by Nishizuka and his colleagues since 1980 have demonstrated that the liberated 1,2-diacylglycerol acts as a membrane-associated second messenger which activates protein kinase C (8), and more recent studies stimulated by Berridge and Irvine have indicated that inositol 1,4,5-trisphosphate might be a water-soluble second messenger that forms a functional link between receptor activation and the release of Ca^{2+} from a cell-associated pool into the cytosol (10).

This chapter will briefly review the recent evidence that identifies the phosphodiesterase-catalysed breakdown of PtdIns4,5P_2 (and possibly also of phosphatidylinositol 4-phosphate; PtdIns4P) as the initial receptor-controlled step in stimulated inositol lipid metabolism.

II. EARLY STUDIES

In the 1960's, there was no clear indication as to which step(s) in inositol lipid metabolism were controlled by neurotransmitters and other stimuli; the reaction most commonly nominated as a potential control point was the phosphorylation of 1,2-diacylglycerol by diacylglycerol kinase. The first clear statement that the controlled step

was likely to be the phosphodiesterase-catalysed breakdown of
an inositol lipid came from Durell and his colleagues in 1969
(11). They also realised that all of the evidence available
at the time was compatible with receptor-controlled breakdown
of any or all of the three inositol glycerophospholipids
(PtdIns, PtdIns4P and PtdIns4,5P$_2$). The same authors offered
a limited amount of evidence to suggest that inositol
monophosphate and bisphosphate accumulated in stimulated
synaptosomes: this pointed to hydrolysis either of PtdIns and
PtdIns4P or of polyphosphoinositides (followed by sequential
dephosphorylation of the released inositol bis- and/or
trisphosphates). After this, PtdIns4P and PtdIns4,5P$_2$ were
largely ignored for many years, partly because the most commonly used methods for lipid extraction and analysis leave
them as unexamined components associated with the tissue residue and partly because the dominant ideas of the 1970's placed
emphasis on 'PtdIns breakdown' rather than upon changes in
PtdIns4P and PtdIns4,5P$_2$ metabolism.

Attention was redirected to PtdIns4P and PtdIns4,5P$_2$ in
the late 1970's, when several laboratories (including those of
Buckley, Lester, Abdel-Latif, Michell, Hawthorne, and
Schanberg) observed rapid changes in the metabolism of these
lipids in perturbed cells. In particular there was rapid
breakdown of these lipids when cytoplasmic Ca^{2+} concentrations
were raised to 'pathological' levels (for a review, see ref.
12). At this time, Hawthorne and Pickard (13) also reiterated
Durell's earlier statement that the existing information was
explicable in terms of stimulated breakdown of any of the inositol lipids, even though there was still no convincing evidence that a lipid other than PtdIns was likely to be the
substrate of receptor-controlled phosphodiesterase activity.
However, a substantial body of information has accumulated
since 1980 that appears to demonstrate, beyond reasonable
doubt, that Ca^{2+}-mobilizing receptors stimulate the hydrolysis
of PtdIns4,5P$_2$ to 1,2-diacylglycerol and inositol
1,4,5-trisphosphate. Whether this is the only reaction that
is activated by receptors is still uncertain; receptors might
also control PtdIns4P hydrolysis, but it now seems unlikely
that there is any direct control of PtdIns hydrolysis.

III. RECEPTOR-STIMULATED INOSITOL LIPID METABOLISM
IN HEPATOCYTES

Between 1977 and 1980 it was established that isolated rat
liver cells constitute an excellent experimental system in
which to analyse the relationships between stimulation of
Ca^{2+}-mobilizing receptors and cellular responses, including

stimulated inositol lipid metabolism (14-18). As a result of
these and subsequent studies, we now know that rat hepatocytes
possess at least five types of receptors that function in this
way: these respond to α_1-adrenergic stimuli, vasopressin
(acting at V_1-receptors), angiotensin, ATP (and possibly other
adenine nucleotides) and 1-0-alkyl-2-acetyl-sn-glyceryl-3-
phosphorylcholine (also known as AGEPC, platelet activating
factor or PAF) (14-28).   Receptors that work through other
mechanisms, sometimes involving control of adenylate cyclase,
do not produce this response: ineffective receptors in hepatocytes include those that respond to insulin, α_2- and
β-adrenergic stimuli, prolactin, glucagon and oestradiol.
        Receptor-controlled changes in inositol lipid metabolism
in hepatocytes were initially analysed as changes in the
labelling of PtdIns (14-18), as an increased rate of turnover
of prelabelled PtdIns (16,18,19) and as a net depletion of
cellular PtdIns on stimulation (16,19).   The only comment on
PtdIns4P and PtdIns4,5P$_2$ in these early papers stated that
their labelling was unchanged after prolonged stimulation
(17).   In 1980, we embarked on a study of the possible rapid
effects of Ca^{2+}-mobilizing stimuli on the metabolism of
PtdIns4P and PtdIns4,5P$_2$ in hepatocytes, in the mistaken
belief that the receptor-controlled elevation of cytosol Ca^{2+}
concentration in these cells would cause activation of a
Ca^{2+}-controlled polyphosphoinositide phosphodiesterase similar
to that present in the plasma membrane of erythrocytes
(29,20).   As expected, we observed a very rapid receptor-
stimulated breakdown of PtdIns4P and PtdIns4,5P$_2$ but it soon
became apparent that this was not a consequence of the
receptor-activated rise in cytosol Ca^{2+} concentration (21,23).
Moreover, extension of our earlier studies of the
polyphosphoinositide phosphodiesterase of the erythrocyte
indicated clearly that this enzyme was unlikely to be
controlled by the changes in cytosol Ca^{2+} concentration that
occur in response to physiological stimulation of healthy
cells (30).

IV. RAPID METABOLIC TURNOVER OF PtdIns4P AND PtdIns4,5P$_2$ IN UNSTIMULATED HEPATOCYTES

        PtdIns is usually present in mammalian cells as around 10%
of the total membrane phospholipid, making it relatively ame-
nable to quantitative analysis by chemical methods.   However,
PtdIns4P and PtdIns4,5P$_2$ are generally present at much lower
concentrations, so that it is difficult to detect changes in
their concentrations by these methods: in liver cells they
comprise less than 5% of the total inositol lipids (23,27).

It is therefore easier to pre-label cells with ^{32}P or ^{3}H-inositol, and then to assess changes in the labelling of PtdIns4P and PtdIns4,5P$_2$ that occur on stimulation. If these changes are to be interpreted as a reflection of changes in the concentrations of the lipids, then these two lipids must come to isotopic equilibrium with PtdIns and the γ-phosphate of ATP, their two immediate metabolic precursors, before application of a stimulus. There is also a potential ambiguity inherent in studies using ^{32}P, in that PtdIns4,5P$_2$ possesses three phosphate groups, each of which turns over independently; the phosphodiester group comes directly from PtdIns and labels relatively slowly, whereas the 4-phosphate and 5-phosphate are donated by ATP and turn over rapidly.

We have recently devised simple methods for analysing separately the 1-, 4- and 5-phosphate groups of PtdIns4,5P$_2$ (and also the 1- and 4-phosphates of PtdIns4P)(31). These methods have been used, together with a new and simplified method for determining the specific radioactivity of the γ-phosphate of ATP (32), to follow the kinetics of labelling of PtdIns4P and PtdIns4,5P$_2$ in hepatocytes after the addition of [^{32}P]-P$_i$. Fig. 1a shows the labelling of the γ-phosphate of hepatocyte ATP, which is also included (as the dashed line) with curves describing the labelling of the monoester phosphate groups of PtdIns4P and PtdIns4,5P$_2$ in Figs. 1b and 1c: for simplicity, the labelling of the two monoester phosphate groups of PtdIns4,5P$_2$ has been presented as a composite figure. It is clear that the labelling of these monoesterified phosphate groups only lags slightly behind the labelling of the γ-phosphate of ATP. We cannot derive accurate estimates of the turnover rates of the 4-phosphate of PtdIns4P and the 5-phosphate of PtdIns4,5P$_2$ from these data, since the labelling kinetics of ATP and the lipids are not temporally resolved to a sufficient extent. However, an inevitable deduction from this observation is that the two kinase/phosphatase cycles responsible for the turnover of these phosphate groups (Scheme 1) must operate at a very high rate even in unstimulated hepatocytes, so achieving the turnover of the cellular pools of PtdIns4P and PtdIns4,5P$_2$ every

Scheme 1

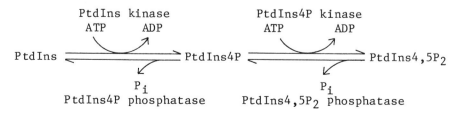

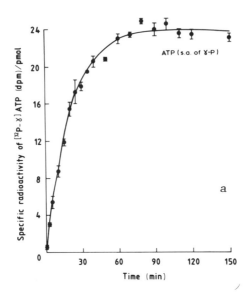

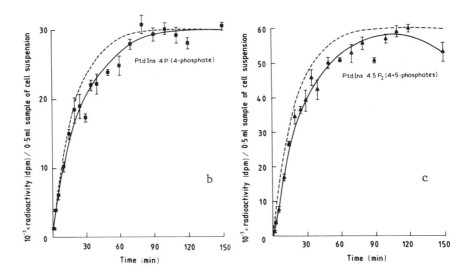

FIGURE 1. Time-course of the labelling of the γ-phosphate of (a) ATP and of the monoester phosphate groups of (b) PtdIns4P and (c) PtdIns4,5P$_2$ in rat hepatocytes. Cells were incubated in ^{32}P-free medium, before addition of ^{32}P-P$_i$ at t=0. The incubation conditions and analytical methods were as described in refs. 23, 31 & 32.

few minutes (or even more rapidly). This process will entail the continuous consumption of an appreciable quantity of ATP simply to maintain the concentrations of these two lipids at relatively constant concentrations, so it seems likely that it is of some value to the cell for this to occur.

V. Ca^{2+}-MOBILIZING STIMULI DECREASE THE STEADY-STATE CONCENTRATIONS OF PtdIns4P AND PtdIns4,5P$_2$ IN HEPATOCYTES

The monoester phosphate groups of PtdIns4P and PtdIns4,5P$_2$ appear to be close to isotopic equilibrium with the γ-phosphate of ATP, their immediate isotopic precursor, within about 60–80 min of the addition of ^{32}P-P$_i$ (Fig. 1). If a high concentration of a Ca^{2+}-mobilizing stimulus (vasopressin, angiotensin, α$_1$-adrenergic, ATP or AGEPC) is added at that time, then there is a very rapid decrease in the labelling of PtdIns4,5P$_2$ and, usually to a lesser degree, of PtdIns4P: an example of such a response is shown in Fig. 2. The initial rate at which this decrease occurs represents a depletion of cellular PtdIns4,5P$_2$ at about one per cent per second. A new steady-state concentration is achieved within about 1 min, usually at 50–90% of the concentration established before application of the stimulus. That this is

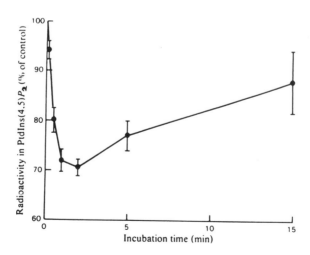

FIGURE 2. Rapid vasopressin-stimulated depletion of PtdIns4,5P$_2$ in rat liver cells. 230 nM vasopressin was added to ^{32}P-labelled cells at t=0. For experimental details, see ref. 23.

indeed a new steady state, rather than cessation of
PtdIns4,5P$_2$ breakdown because of receptor desensitization, is
established by the observation that stimulation continues to
liberate inositol phosphates from lipids even after the concentration of PtdIns4,5P$_2$ passes its nadir (see later).

Detailed studies of receptor-controlled PtdIns4,5P$_2$
depletion in hepatocytes have indicated that it has the
following characteristics (23,26-28). The response to each of
the five Ca^{2+}-mobilizing stimuli mentioned above is probably
mediated by a separate class of cell-surface receptor.
PtdIns4,5P$_2$ depletion can be detected within a few seconds of
the addition of a stimulus, i.e. over a time-scale similar to
that involved in the receptor-controlled rise in cytosol Ca^{2+}
concentration and activation of glycogen phosphorylase in the
same cells. At least for vasopressin and angiotensin, there
is a close quantitative correlation between occupation of
receptors by agonist molecules and activation of PtdIns4,5P$_2$
breakdown, whereas only a small proportion of the total receptor population needs to be activated in order to raise the
cytosol Ca^{2+} concentration enough to fully activate glycogen
phosphorylase (23,27). Despite this distinction between the
dose-response relationships for activation of PtdIns4,5P$_2$
breakdown and of glycogen phosphorylase a substantial fraction
of the PtdIns4,5P$_2$ breakdown response survives a protocol of
cellular Ca^{2+} deprivation that is sufficiently severe to abolish the activation of phosphorylase (23,27). More vigorous
Ca^{2+} deprivation does abolish the receptor-activated depletion of PtdIns4,5P$_2$, but this does not indicate, contrary to
the conclusion reached by Rhodes et al. (26), that the
receptor-induced rise in cytosol Ca^{2+} concentration controls
PtdIns4,5P$_2$ breakdown. It seems more likely, as first pointed
out some years ago (3), that the phosphodiesterase responsible
for receptor-stimulated breakdown of PtdIns4,5P$_2$ is an enzyme
that requires Ca^{2+}, but that the quantities of Ca^{2+} in unstimulated cells (approximately 0.1 - 0.2 μM in hepatocytes; refs.
33,34) are sufficient to satisfy this requirement. Hence the
available evidence indicates that the receptor-stimulated
increase in cytosol Ca^{2+} concentration plays no role in the
control of this reaction.

VI. ACCUMULATION OF INOSITOL PHOSPHATES
IN STIMULATED HEPATOCYTES

Although the results summarized above strongly suggest
that activation of Ca^{2+}-mobilizing receptors activates a
phosphodiesterase-catalysed breakdown of PtdIns4,5P$_2$ (see ref.
23 for a detailed discussion of this interpretation), they do

not unambiguously establish the occurrence of this reaction. Other observations, including the transient appearance of 1,2-diacylglycerol and of newly synthesized ^{32}P-labelled phosphatidate, have for many years pointed to the participation of a phosphodiesterase in receptor-activated inositol lipid metabolism (1,11), but they have given no indication which inositol lipid was the target of the activated phosphodiesterase.

Recent studies, the first of which were by Berridge, Downes and their colleagues, have demonstrated that inositol trisphosphate and bisphosphate are the earliest detectable products of receptor-stimulated inositol lipid breakdown, at least in blowfly and rat salivary glands and in rat brain (35,36). We have undertaken similar studies with rat hepatocytes. Cells were labelled with ^{3}H-inositol and excess labelled inositol 'chased' out of the cells (both stages were in the presence of 0.1 mM total inositol). The cells were then stimulated with a maximally effective concentration of vasopressin. Li$^+$ was included in the incubations in order to inhibit inositol 1-phosphate phosphatase and hence preserve any liberated inositol phosphates (37,38). During stimula-

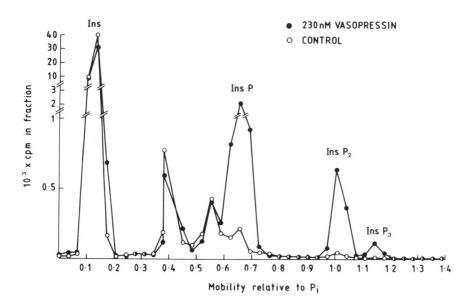

FIGURE 3. Accumulation of labelled inositol phosphates in ^{3}H-inositol-labelled rat hepatocytes incubated in 10 mM Li$^+$ and stimulated for 10 min with 230 nM vasopressin. Acid-soluble aqueous fractions from control and vasopressin-stimulated cells were subjected to high-voltage electrophoresis by the technique of Dawson and Clarke (42).

tion, there was a substantial accumulation of polar and
^{3}H-labelled material. Analysis of the products by high-
voltage electrophoresis and anion-exchange chromatography
revealed that after 10 min of stimulation a small fraction of
the released radioactivity was in inositol trisphosphate, with
the remainder distributed between inositol bisphosphate and
inositol monophosphate (Fig. 3). Other polar metabolites of
inositol, which eluted from ion-exchange columns with inositol
monophosphate, were also present. However, these were
resolved from inositol monophosphate by high-voltage
electrophoresis: these compounds were not degraded by
alkaline phosphatase and their concentrations were unchanged
by stimulation, so we suspect that they are produced by
metabolism of inositol through some route unrelated to lipids
(e.g. inositol oxidation).

    Accumulation of inositol phosphates started immediately
upon addition of vasopressin to hepatocytes, and continued for
at least 15 min (Fig. 4). As noted above, the concentrations
of PtdIns4P and PtdIns4,5P$_2$ change only slowly after the first
minute of stimulation (Fig. 2), so this continued production
of inositol phosphates must involve a striking increase in the
metabolic flux of ^{3}H-inositol, via PtdIns, PtdIns4P and
PtdIns4,5P$_2$, into water-soluble inositol phosphates. Indeed,
the rate of appearance of inositol phosphates in these in-
tensely stimulated cells represents the breakdown of at least
one percent of the inositol lipids in the cells every minute,
a figure that is in remarkable agreement with our previous
measurements of the rate of depletion of PtdIns in
vasopressin-stimulated hepatocytes (19).

    We included Li$^+$ ions in our assays because they are known
effectively to inhibit inositol 1-phosphate phosphatase.
However, we have also observed that Li$^+$ at high concentrations
changes the relative quantities of the different inositol
phosphates that accumulate in stimulated cells. At 50 mM Li$^+$,
which produces no change in the receptor-activated fall in the
steady-state concentrations of PtdIns4P and PtdIns4,5P$_2$ on
stimulation, about 15% of the total water-soluble phosphates
accumulate as inositol trisphosphate, as compared with less
than 5% in cells stimulated in the presence of 1 mM Li$^+$ (S.
Palmer and P. T. Hawkins, unpublished data).

    It is possible that activation of Ca^{2+}-mobilizing recep-
tors stimulates phosphodiesterase-catalysed breakdown of more
than one inositol phospholipid, but if only a single reaction
is the target of the receptor-controlled phosphodiesterase
then the presence of inositol trisphosphate amongst the cellular products of that process identifies that lipid as
PtdIns4,5P$_2$. We would suggest, in the continued absence of a
specific inhibitor of inositol 1,4,5-trisphosphate 5-phospha-
tase, that the best method that is currently available for

investigation of the characteristics of receptor-controlled PtdIns4,5P$_2$ breakdown in liver cells is analysis of the inositol phosphates that accumulate in cells stimulated in the presence of a high concentration of Li$^+$ ions.

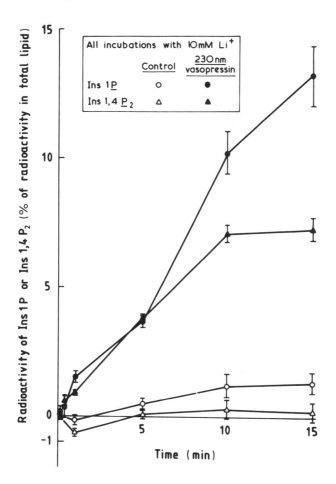

FIGURE 4. Time-course of accumulation of ^{3}H-labelled inositol monophosphate and bisphosphate in vasopressin-stimulated hepatocytes. Incubation conditions were as in Fig. 3, and accumulated inositol phosphates were separated by ion-exchange chromatography essentially as in ref. 29. The amounts of accumulated inositol trisphosphate were too small to be reliably estimated by this method, and are therefore omitted. The amounts of inositol phosphates accumulated are expressed by reference to the total amount of ^{3}H-inositol present in hepatocyte lipids at the time of addition of vasopressin.

Table I. Stimuli That Provoke Breakdown of PtdIns4,5P$_2$, as Indicated Either by PtdIns4,5P$_2$, Depletion or Inositol Trisphosphate Accumulation.

Stimulus	Cell or Tissue	Evidence for: PtdIns4,5P$_2$ depletion	InsP$_3$ accumulation
Muscarinic cholinergic	Synaptosomes		11
	Iris muscle	43	43
	Exocrine pancreas	45	
	Parotid gland	40	35, 44
	Lacrimal gland	46	
	Brain		35
α$_1$-Adrenergic	Iris muscle	43	43
	Liver	23,26,27	
	Parotid gland	40	35
	Lacrimal gland	46	
	Brain		35
V$_1$-Vasopressin	Liver	3, 23	
	Sympathetic ganglia		see text
	Hippocampus		58
	Adipocytes		L. Stephens & S. Logan R. Rubio & P. Newsholme
Angiotensin	Liver	23	
Substance P	Parotid gland	40	

Table I. Stimuli That Provoke Breakdown of PtdIns4,5P$_2$, as Indicated Either by PtdIns4,5P$_2$, Depletion or Inositol Trisphosphate Accumulation. (Continued)

Stimulus	Cell or Tissue	Evidence for:	
		PtdIns4,5P$_2$ Depletion	InsP$_3$ accumulation
Pancreozymin	Exocrine pancreas	45	
5-Hydroxytryptamine	Fly salivary gland	36	35
TRH	GH3 cells	47-50	47-50
fmet-leu-phe	Neutrophils	51	
Thrombin	Platelets	52	53
ADP	Platelets	54	
AGEPC (PAF-acether)	Platelets	55-57	
	Liver	28	
Concanavalin A	T lymphocytes	T. Sasaki	
TSH	Thyroid cells	L. Kohn	

Sources of information are indicated by reference number. When the information is from a personal communication, then the name of the author communicating the information is given.

VII. STIMULATED PtdIns4,5P$_2$ HYDROLYSIS: A WIDESPREAD
RECEPTOR-ACTIVATED EVENT?

The evidence summarized above clearly indicates that
PtdIns hydrolysis is an important receptor-activated event in
stimulated hepatocytes, but it does not indicate whether this
reaction is likely to be of similar significance in other
cells. However, we have always been of the opinion that the
reaction responsible for initiating stimulated inositol lipid
metabolism is likely to be the same in all situations, whatever the combination of tissue and stimulus being considered
(1-3,39). When we obtained our first results indicating that
receptors control PtdIns4,5P$_2$ hydrolysis in hepatocytes, we
suggested that this type of phosphodiesterase-catalyzed breakdown of PtdIns4,5P$_2$ might be the initiating step in information transmission in all situations in which receptors operate
by controlling inositol lipid breakdown (3). The first con-
firmation of this view came from Berridge and Putney and their
respective colleagues (35,36,40). More recently, there have
been many more studies that point to the same conclusion:
these are summarized in Table I. As a result of these studies
it now seems likely that activation of Ca^{2+}-mobilizing
receptors, of whatever type, always stimulates a phosphodiesterase that attacks PtdIns4,5P$_2$, and possibly also
PtdIns4P. Figure 5 presents a schematic summary of the way in
which activation of this reaction may lead to all of the
changes in inositol lipid and inositol phosphate metabolism
that are known to follow receptor activation.
   The subcellular site, enzymic characteristics and mechanism of activation of the phosphodiesterase responsible for
this reaction are at present unknown, and their analysis must
provide a major focus of research activity over the next few
years. At present there are two candidates for this role.
Perhaps most plausible is the idea that receptors exert relatively direct control (perhaps involving a guanine nucleotide-
requiring coupling component?) over a plasma membrane-bound
phosphodiesterase that is similar to the enzyme found in
erythrocytes from several species (29,30). However, Irvine
and his colleagues have recently found that a so-called
'PtdIns phosphodiesterase', which has long been known as a
component of the cytosol of many cells, also behaves as an
excellent PtdIns4,5P$_2$ phosphodiesterase when assayed under
conditions approximating to those that might prevail in the
cytosol of a stimulated cell (41). Indeed, the enzymic
characteristics of the cytoplasmic and membrane-associated
activities appear remarkably similar when they are both
assayed under these conditions, thus raising the possibility
that they represent two forms of the same enzyme species.

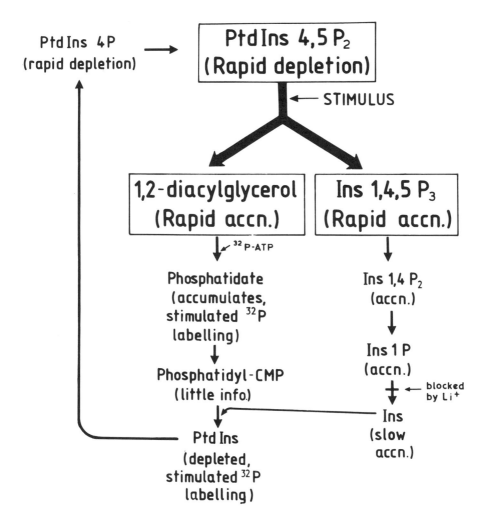

FIGURE 5. A scheme to suggest how the various changes in lipid metabolism that are normally encompassed within 'the PtdIns response' may all be either direct or indirect results of receptor-stimulated hydrolysis of PtdIns4,5P$_2$ by a phospho-diesterase.

VIII. WHAT IS THE FUNCTION OF RECEPTOR–STIMULATED PtdIns4,5P$_2$ HYDROLYSIS?

The idea that receptor–stimulated breakdown of inositol phospholipid(s) might be an essential coupling step that lies between activation of receptors and a rise in cytoplasmic Ca^{2+} concentration was first mooted in 1975 (1), but without any clear proposal as to how this mobilization of Ca^{2+} might be achieved. As soon as it was realized that receptors control a rapid breakdown of PtdIns4,5P$_2$, there were suggestions that the mobilized Ca^{2+} might come from a pool bound to the headgroups of PtdIns4,5P$_2$ at the inner face of the plasma membrane (e.g. ref. 42). Such ideas appear to be ruled out by the fact that Ca^{2+} is mobilized in substantial molar excess over the degraded lipid (see refs. 23,27, for other arguments against this type of model). A very exciting recent development is the idea that inositol trisphosphate might act as an intracellular messenger that releases Ca^{2+} from an intracellular store, possibly in the endoplasmic reticulum (10), but final judgment on this idea will have to await further information.

The idea that the 1,2–diacylglycerol, the other product of PtdIns4,5P$_2$ hydrolysis, may be a second messenger responsible for the activation of protein kinase C is discussed by Nishizuka elsewhere in this book.

IX. CONCLUSION

It seems likely that recent studies have finally identified phosphodiesterase–catalysed hydrolysis of PtdIns4,5P$_2$, yielding 1,2–diacylglycerol and inositol 1,4,5–trisphosphate, as the first biochemical event to be initiated by a diverse family of cell–surface receptors that respond to hormones, neurotransmitters, growth factors, antigens and other cellular stimuli. The two products of this reaction may both have important functions as second messengers. Future studies must determine the mechanisms by which receptors control PtdIns4,5P$_2$ hydrolysis and by which these novel second messengers exert control over their intracellular targets.

REFERENCES

1. Michell, R. H., Biochim. Biophys. Acta 415:81 (1975).
2. Michell, R. H., Trends Biochem. Sci. 4:128 (1979).
3. Michell, R. H., Kirk, C. J., Jones, L. M., Downes, C. P., and Creba, J. A., Phil. Trans. Roy. Soc., Series B. 296:123 (1981).
4. Berridge, M. J., Trends Pharmacol. Sci. 1:419 (1980).
5. Berridge, M. J., Mol. Cell. Endocrinol. 24:115 (1981).
6. Irvine, R. F., Dawson, R. M. C., and Freinkel, N., in "Contemporary Metabolism, Volume 2" (N. Freinkel, ed.), p.301. Plenum Press, New York, 1982.
7. Fain, J. N., in "Hormone Receptors" (L. Kohn, ed.), p.237. John Wiley, Chichester, 1982.
8. Nishizuka, Y., Trends Biochem. Sci. 8:13 (1983).
9. Michell, R. H., and Lapetina, E. G., Nature 240:104 (1972).
10. Streb, H., Irvine, R. F., Berridge, M. J., and Schulz, I., Nature 306:67 (1983).
11. Durell, J., Garland, J. T., and Friedel, R. O., Science 165:862 (1969).
12. Downes, C. P., and Michell, R. H., Cell Calcium 3:467 (1982).
13. Hawthorne, J. N., and Pickard, M. R., J. Neurochem. 32:5 (1975).
14. Kirk, C. J., Verrinder, T. R., and Hems, D. A., FEBS Lett. 83:267 (1977).
15. Kirk, C. J., Rodrigues, L. M., and Hems, D. A., Biochem. J. 178:493 (1979).
16. Billah, M. M., and Michell, R. H., Biochem. J. 182:661 (1979).
17. Tolbert, M. E. M., White, A. C., Aspry, K., Cutts, J., and Fain, J. N., J. Biol. Chem. 255:1938 (1980).
18. Michell, R. H., Kirk, C. J., and Billah, M. M., Biochem. Soc. Trans. 7:861 (1979).
19. Kirk, C. J., Michell, R. H., and Hems, D. A., Biochem. J. 194:155 (1981).
20. Michell, R. H., in "Lipoprotein Metabolism and Endocrine Regulation" (L. W. Hessel, and H. M. J. Krans, eds.), p.203. Elsevier, Amsterdam, 1979.
21. Kirk, C. J., Cell Calcium 3:399 (1982).
22. Takenawa, T., Homma, Y., and Nagai, Y., Biochem. Pharmacol. 31:2663 (1982).
23. Creba, J. A., Downes, C. P., Hawkins, P. T., Brewster, G., Michell, R. H., and Kirk, C. J., Biochem. J. 212:733 (1983).
24. Prpic, V., Blackmore, P. F., and Exton, J. H., J. Biol. Chem. 257:11315 (1982).

25. Prpic, V., Blackmore, P. F., and Exton, J. H., J. Biol. Chem. 257:11323 (1982).
26. Rhodes, D., Prpic, V., Exton, J. H., and Blackmore, P. F., J. Biol. Chem. 258:2770 (1983).
27. Thomas, A. P., Marks, J. S., Coll, K. E., and Williamson, J. R., J. Biol. Chem. 258:5716 (1983).
28. Shukla, S. D., Buxton, D. B., Olson, M. S., and Hanahan, D. J., J. Biol. Chem. 258:10212 (1983).
29. Downes, C. P., and Michell, R. H., Biochem. J. 198:133 (1981).
30. Downes, C. P., and Michell, R. H., Biochem. J. 202:53 (1982).
31. Hawkins, P. T., Michell, R. H., and Kirk, C. J., Biochem. J. 218:785 (1984).
32. Hawkins, P. T., Michell, R. H., and Kirk, C. J., Biochem. J. 210:717 (1983).
33. Williamson, J. R., Cooper, R. H., and Hoek, J. B., Biochim. Biophys. Acta 639:243 (1981).
34. Blackmore, P. F., Hughes, B. P., Charest, R., Shuman, E. A., and Exton, J. H., J. Biol. Chem. 258:10488 (1983).
35. Berridge, M. J., Dawson, R. M. C., Downes, C. P., Heslop, J. P., and Irvine, R. F., Biochem. J. 212:473 (1983).
36. Berridge, M. J., Biochem. J. 212:849 (1983).
37. Hallcher, L. M., and Sherman, W. R., J. Biol. Chem. 255:10896 (1980).
38. Berridge, M. J., Downes, C. P., and Hanley, M. R., Biochem. J. 206:587 (1982).
39. Lapetina, E. G., and Michell, R. H., FEBS Lett. 31:1 (1973).
40. Weiss, S. J., McKinney, J., and Putney, J. W., Biochem. J. 206:555 (1982).
41. Irvine, R. F., Biochem. J. 218:177 (1984).
42. Dawson, R. M. C., and Clarke, R., Biochem. J. 127:113 (1972).
43. Abdel-Latif, A. A., Handbook of Neurochemistry 3:91 (1983).
44. Downes, C. P., and Wusteman, M. M., Biochem. J. 216:633 (1983).
45. Putney, J. W., Burgess, G. M., Halenda, S. P., McKinney, J. S., and Rubin, R. P., Biochem. J. 212:483 (1983).
46. Godfrey, P. P., and Putney, J. W., Biochem. J. 218:187 (1983).
47. Macphee, C. H., and Drummond, A. H., Mol. Pharmacol. 25:193 (1984).
48. Drummond, A. H., Bushfield, M., and Macphee, C. H., Mol. Pharmacol. 25:201 (1984).
49. Rebecchi, M. J., and Gershengorn, M. C., Biochem. J. 216:299 (1983).
50. Martin, T. F. J., J. Biol. Chem. 258:14816 (1983).

51. Volpi, M., Yassin, R., Naccache, P. H., and Sha'afi, R. I., Biochem. Biophys. Res. Commun. 112:957 (1982).
52. Billah, M. M., and Lapetina, E. G., J. Biol. Chem. 257:12705 (1982).
53. Agranoff, B. W., Murphy, P., and Seguin, E. B., J. Biol. Chem. 258:2076 (1983).
54. Vickers, J. D., Kinlough-Rathbone, R. L., and Mustard, J. F., Blood, 60:1247 (1982).
55. Lapetina, E. G., J. Biol. Chem. 257:7314 (1982).
56. Shukla, S. D., and Hanahan, D. J., Arch. Biochem. Biophys. 227:626 (1983).
57. Mauco, G., Chap, H., and Douste-Blazy, L., FEBS Lett. 153:361 (1983).
58. Bone, E. A., Fretten, P., Palmer, S., Kirk, C. J., and Michell, R. H., Biochem. J. (in press) (1984).

CALCIUM MOBILIZATION AND PHOSPHOLIPID DEGRADATION IN SIGNAL TRANSDUCTION[1]

K. Kaibuchi,
M. Sawamura
Y. Katakami
U. Kikkawa
Y. Takai
Y. Nishizuka

Department of Biochemistry
Kobe University School of Medicine
Kobe

and

Department of Cell Biology
National Institute for Basic Biology
Okazaki

I. OVERVIEW

Inositol phospholipid turnover provoked by a wide variety of biologically active substances appears to be linked directly to protein phosphorylation through activation of a novel protein kinase (protein kinase C). This protein phosphorylation is a prerequisite for transmembrane control of

---

[1]This investigation has been supported in part by research grants from the Research Fund of the Ministry of Education, Science and Culture, the Intractable Diseases Division, Public Health Bureau, the Ministry of Health and Welfare, a Grant-in-Aid of New Drug Development from the Ministry of Health and Welfare, the Science and Technology Agency, the Yamanouchi Foundation for Research on Metabolic Disorders and the Mitsuhisa Cancer Research Foundation, Japan.

cellular functions and proliferation, and evidence is available that the receptor-linked activation of this protein kinase and Ca^{2+} mobilization act synergistically to elicit full physiological cellular responses. Tumor-promoting phorbol esters are intercalated into the membrane phospholipid bilayer and directly activate protein kinase C without inducing inositol phospholipid turnover.

II. INTRODUCTION

It is generally accepted that various peptide hormones, neurotransmitters, growth factors and many other biologically active substances provoke inositol phospholipid turnover in their target tissues. In a manner as yet unknown this phospholipid turnover is usually associated with Ca^{2+} mobilization with few exceptions (1). Originally, phosphatidylinositol was proposed to be broken down upon stimulation of the receptors (2), but recent evidence suggests that phosphatidylinositol bisphosphate is more likely the immediate target for the signal-induced degradation of inositol phospholipids, even though this phospholipid is a very minor component in membranes (see for a review ref. 3). More recently, Streb et al. (4) have postulated that inositol triphosphate, one of the earliest products of phosphatidylinositol bisphosphate breakdown, may act as an intracellular mediator of Ca^{2+} mobilization, but this attractive hypothesis is yet to be explored further. On the other hand, diacylglycerol that is another early product has been found in this laboratory to serve as an activator of protein kinase C (Ca^{2+}-activated, phospholipid-dependent protein kinase) which appears to play a crucial role in the transmembrane control of cellular functions and proliferation (5-9). A proposed pathway of this signal transduction is outlined in Fig. 1. This article will briefly describe evidence of the link of inositol phospholipid turnover to the protein phosphorylation, and its synergistic role with Ca^{2+} in eliciting full cellular responses. The direct action of tumor-promoting phorbol esters on this signal transduction will also be described.

III. ACTIVATION OF PROTEIN KINASE C

At a physiological concentration of Ca^{2+}, protein kinase C requires diacylglycerol in addition to phospholipid. Diacylglycerol is normally almost absent from membranes but is transiently produced from inositol phospholipids in a signal-

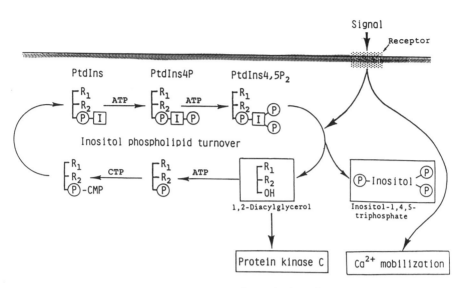

FIGURE 1. A proposed mechanism of signal transduction. PtdIns, phosphatidylinositol; PtdIns4P, phosphatidylinositol monophosphate; PtdIns4,5P$_2$, phosphatidylinositol bisphosphate; R$_1$ and R$_2$, fatty acyl groups; I, inositol; and P, phosphoryl group.

dependent manner. Kinetically, a small quantity of diacylglycerol dramatically increases the affinity of protein kinase C for Ca^{2+}, and renders this enzyme fully active without a net increase in the Ca^{2+} concentration (5-7). Thus, it is worth noting for later discussion that the activation of this protein kinase is a biologically Ca^{2+}-independent process, because its sensitivity to Ca^{2+} is greatly modulated by the signal-induced breakdown of inositol phospholipids. Evidence to support this view has primarily come from a series of experiments with platelets as a test cell system, since many agonists and antagonists for the aggregation and release reactions are known.

When platelets are stimulated by thrombin or collagen, two endogenous proteins having molecular weights of 40,000 (40K protein) and 20,000 (20K protein) are rapidly and heavily phosphorylated, and the phosphorylation of these proteins is associated with release reactions (10-13). The 20K protein is myosin light chain (14), and the calmodulin-dependent phosphorylation of this protein requires mobilization of

Ca^{2+} (15). It has been described earlier (13) that the 40K
protein isolated from human platelets serves as a substrate
for protein kinase C, and the signal-induced formation of
endogenous diacylglycerol always accompanies the 40K protein
phosphorylation as schematically shown in Fig. 2. Preceding
reports (16,17) have also shown that tumor-promoting phorbol
esters such as 12-O-tetradecanoylphorbol-13-acetate (TPA) and
phorbol-12,13-dibutyrate can substitute for diacylglycerol and
directly activate protein kinase C in the presence of Ca^{2+} and
phospholipid.

In cell-free systems various diacylglycerols are equally
capable of activating protein kinase C (18). On the other
hand, in intact cell systems, diacylglycerols containing two
long fatty acyl moieties such as diolein cannot be intercalated into the membrane. However, if one long fatty acyl
moiety is replaced by an acetyl group, then the resulting
diacylglycerol, 1-oleoyl-2-acetylglycerol, appears to gain
detergent-like properties and to activate protein kinase C
directly without interaction with cell surface receptors.

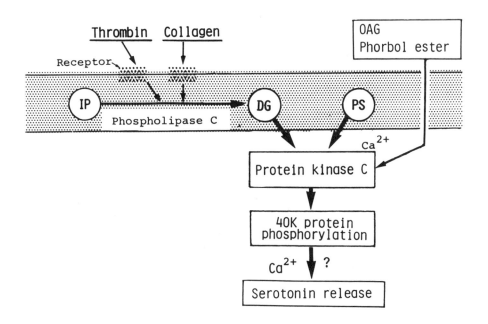

FIGURE 2. Schematic representation of inositol phospholipid degradation, 40K protein phosphorylation, and serotonin
release in platelets. IP, inositol phospholipids; DG,
diacylglycerol; PS, phosphatidylserine; and OAG, 1-oleoyl-2-
acetyl-glycerol.

There is no sign of damage of cell membranes. In the experiments given in Fig. 3, this synthetic diacylglycerol is shown to induce rapid phosphorylation of the 40K protein in platelets just as it is by natural extracellular messengers such as thrombin. Under these conditions neither the breakdown of inositol phospholipids nor the formation of endogenous diacylglycerol is observed. The fingerprint analysis of tryptic phosphopeptides of the radioactive 40K protein preparations indicates that protein kinase C is responsible

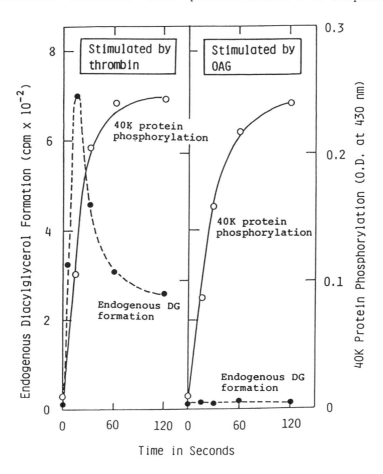

FIGURE 3. Phosphorylation of 40K protein and formation of endogenous diacylglycerol in human platelets stimulated by synthetic diacylglycerol and thrombin. Human platelets were labeled with either [^{3}H]arachidonate or ^{32}Pi, and then stimulated by 1-oleoyl-2-acetyl-glycerol or by thrombin at 37°C for various periods of time indicated. Detailed conditions are described elsewhere (9).

for the observed phosphorylation of the 40K protein in the platelet which is stimulated by synthetic diacylglycerol. Essentially similar results are obtained with TPA in place of synthetic diacylglycerol (16,17).

These results seem to indicate that, in platelets, the receptor-mediated breakdown of inositol phospholipids, either phosphatidylinositol or its bisphosphate, may be directly linked to the activation of protein kinase C, and that synthetic diacylglycerols as well as tumor-promoting phorbol esters can be intercalated into intact cell membranes and activate this protein kinase directly. It is important to emphasize that the activation of this enzyme per se is not related to Ca^{2+} mobilization.

IV. SYNERGISTIC ACTION WITH CALCIUM ION

In general, stimulation of the receptors which provoke inositol phospholipid breakdown mobilizes Ca^{2+}, although there appear to be some exceptions such as bovine adrenal medullary cells (19). A series of experiments with synthetic diacylglycerol and TPA indicates that the activation of protein kinase C alone is only a prerequisite and not a complete requirement for causing full physiological cellular responses. Under appropriate conditions, it is possible to induce protein kinase C activation and Ca^{2+} mobilization independently by the addition of synthetic diacylglycerol or phorbol ester and Ca^{2+} ionophore such as A23187, respectively, as shown in Fig. 4. An advantage to using platelets is the fact that

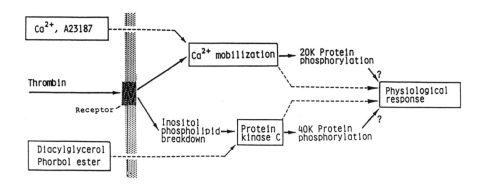

FIGURE 4. Synergistic roles of Ca^{2+} mobilization and protein kinase C activation for serotonin release.

these two events may be selectively quantitated by measuring the phosphorylation of the 40K and 20K proteins mentioned above.

The experiment given in Fig. 5 shows that both protein kinase C activation and Ca^{2+} mobilization are essential and act synergistically to cause the full release of serotonin. It is clear in this experiment that the phosphorylation of 40K protein induced by synthetic diacylglycerol is not enhanced further by the addition of A23187, whereas the overall

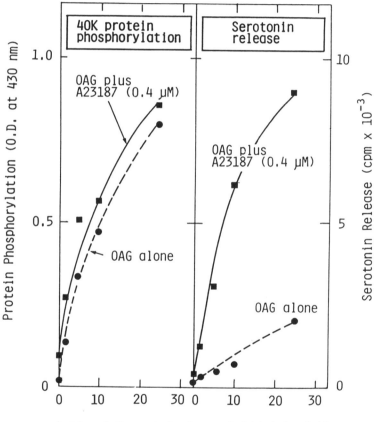

FIGURE 5. Effects of Ca^{2+} ionophore and synthetic diacylglycerol on 40K protein phosphorylation and serotonin release. Human platelets were labeled with either ^{32}Pi or [^{14}C]serotonin, and then stimulated by various concentrations of 1-oleoyl-2-acetyl-glycerol in the presence or absence of A23187 as indicated. Detailed conditions are described elsewhere (9). OAG, 1-oleoyl-2-acetyl-glycerol.

response of platelets is insufficient by the addition of diacylglycerol alone, and the full platelet response may be observed in the simultaneous presence of diacylglycerol and A23187. The Ca^{2+} ionophore alone at the concentration employed shows practically no effect. At higher concentrations such as more than 1 μM, A23187 alone causes significant release of serotonin probably due to a large increase in the Ca^{2+} concentration. A high concentration of Ca^{2+} activates protein kinase C in the absence of diacylglycerol, and presumably also activates phospholipases in a non-specific manner (8,9). Again, similar results are obtained with TPA instead of diacylglycerol (17). However, diacylglycerol and TPA at higher concentrations each causes the release of a significant amount of serotonin in the absence of Ca^{2+} ionophore (8,9,16,17). The reason for this enhanced release is not known, but it is possible that diacylglycerol and TPA may act as membrane fusigens or perturbers and/or as weak Ca^{2+} ionophores by generating superoxide in membranes.

The synergistic effect of synthetic diacylglycerol and Ca^{2+} ionophore is not confined to the serotonin release from platelets. For instance, analogous results are obtained for the lysosomal enzyme release from platelets as well as from neutrophils (20), and also for the histamine release from mast cells (21). Figure 6 shows similar synergistic effects for the growth response in macrophage-depleted peripheral lymphocytes as measured by the radioactive thymidine incorporation into DNA. Both Ca^{2+} ionophore and diacylglycerol or TPA are necessary to bring about the full physiological response. It is noted that the tumor-promoting phorbol ester at low concentrations induces the protein kinase activation alone, and leaves the cell ready to function and proliferate when Ca^{2+} is available. Although the synthetic diacylglycerol exogenously added to platelets is rapidly metabolized in situ to the corresponding phosphatidic acid (9), the tumor promoters are hardly metabolizable and permanently activate protein kinase C.

V. CONCLUSION

The experimental results outlined above have been obtained from the studies of a limited number of selected tissues, mostly platelets. Nevertheless, it is attractive to propose that protein kinase C plays a crucial role in signal transduction for the activation of many cellular functions and proliferation. The evidence thus far available suggests that either the receptor-linked activation of protein kinase C or Ca^{2+} mobilization alone is not sufficient for complete signal

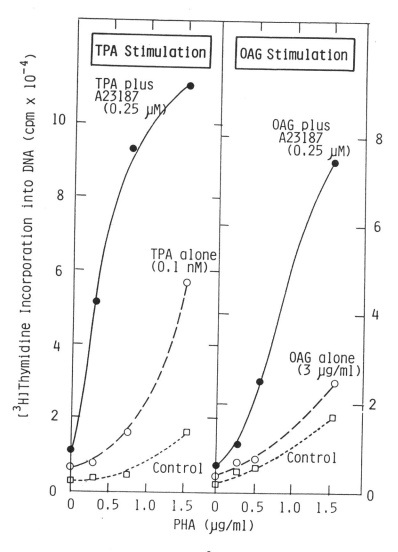

FIGURE 6. Effects of Ca^{2+} ionophore and TPA or synthetic diacylglycerol on phytohemagglutinin-induced DNA synthesis of macrophage-depleted peripheral lymphocytes. Macrophage-depleted peripheral lymphocytes were incubated for 72 hr at 37°C with various concentrations of phytohemagglutinin in the presence or absence of A23187, TPA, and 1-oleoyl-2-acetyl-glycerol as indicated. [^{3}H]Methylthymidine (2 μCi) was added 16 hr before harvesting. Detailed experimental procedures will be described elsewhere. OAG, 1-oleoyl-2-acetyl-glycerol; and PHA, phytohemagglutinin.

transduction, and that their synergistic actions are necessary for the transmembrane control of various cellular processes. Obviously, both Ca^{2+} and protein kinase C may play diverse roles in biological regulation, and the precise targets of protein kinase C will be clarified by further investigations.

ACKNOWLEDGMENTS

We are grateful to Mrs. S. Nishiyama and Mrs. K. Kikkawa for their skillful secretarial assistance.

REFERENCES

1. Michell, R. H., Biochim. Biophys. Acta 415:81 (1975).
2. Hokin, M. R., and Hokin, L. E., J. Biol. Chem. 203:967 (1953).
3. Downes, P., and Michell, R. H., Cell Calcium 3:467 (1982).
4. Streb, H., Irvine, R. F., Berridge, M. J., and Schulz, I., Nature 306:67 (1983).
5. Takai, Y., Kishimoto, A., Kikkawa, U., Mori, T., and Nishizuka, Y., Biochem. Biophys. Res. Commun. 91:1218 (1979).
6. Kishimoto, A., Takai, Y., Mori, T., Kikkawa, U., and Nishizuka, Y., J. Biol. Chem. 255:2273 (1980).
7. Kaibuchi, K., Takai, Y., and Nishizuka, Y., J. Biol. Chem. 256:7146 (1981).
8. Kaibuchi, K., Sano, K., Hoshijima, M., Takai, Y., and Nishizuka, Y., Cell Calcium 3:323 (1982).
9. Kaibuchi, K., Takai, Y., Sawamura, M., Hoshijima, M., Fujikura, T., and Nishizuka, Y., J. Biol. Chem. 258:6761 (1983).
10. Lyons, R. M., Stanford, N., and Majerus, P. W., J. Clin. Invest. 56:924 (1975).
11. Haslam, R. J., and Lynham, J. A., Biochem. Biophys. Res. Commun. 77:714 (1977).
12. Kawahara, Y., Takai, Y., Minakuchi, R., Sano, K., and Nishizuka, Y., Biochem. Biophys. Res. Commun. 97:309 (1980).
13. Sano, K., Takai, Y., Yamanishi, J., and Nishizuka, Y., J. Biol. Chem. 258:2010 (1983).
14. Daniel, J. L., Holmsen, H., and Adelstein, R. S., Thrombos. Haemostas. 38:984 (1977).

15. Yagi, K., Yazawa, M., Kakiuchi, S., Ohshima, M., and Uenishi, K., J. Biol. Chem. 253:1338 (1978).
16. Castagna, M., Takai, Y., Kaibuchi, K., Sano, K., Kikkawa, U., and Nishizuka, Y., J. Biol. Chem. 257:7847 (1982).
17. Yamanishi, J., Takai, Y., Kaibuchi, K., Sano, K., Castagna, M., and Nishizuka, Y., Biochem. Biophys. Res. Commun. 112:778 (1983).
18. Mori, T., Takai, Y., Yu, B., Takahashi, J., Nishizuka, Y., and Fujikura, T., J. Biochem. 91:427 (1982).
19. Swilem, A. M. F., Hawthorne, J. N., and Azila, N., Biochem. Pharmacol. 32: in press (1984).
20. Kajikawa, N., Kaibuchi, K., Matsubara, T., Kikkawa, U., Takai, Y., and Nishizuka, Y., Biochem. Biophys. Res. Commun. 116:743 (1983).
21. Kaibuchi, K., Kikkawa, U., Takai, Y., and Nishizuka, Y., in "Recent Discovered Systems of Enzyme Regulation by Reversible Phosphorylation, Further Advances" (P. Cohen, ed.), p. 81. Elsevier Press, North-Holland, Amsterdam, in press, 1984.

PHOSPHOINOSITIDES, CALCIUM AND SECRETION
IN THE ADRENAL MEDULLA

J. N. Hawthorne
A-M. F. Swilem

Department of Biochemistry
University Hospital and Medical School
Nottingham, U.K.

I. INTRODUCTION

Michell (1) has pointed out that most cell surface receptors associated with the metabolism of phosphoinositides uti-
lise Ca^{2+} as a second messenger. He also suggested that
receptor-linked hydrolysis of these phospholipids caused the
mobilization of Ca^{2+} in the cell, either by opening 'gates'
in the plasma membrane (his original theory, see Fig. 1) or in
more recent modifications of the theory (2) by making this ion
available from intracellular stores.

It has been known for a long time that the hydrolysis of
phosphoinositides[1] by the phospholipase C route (Fig. 2) is
catalysed by a Ca^{2+}-dependent enzyme (3) and so an alternative
explanation of the phosphoinositide effect is that hydrolysis
of these lipids is a consequence, not a cause of increased
cytoplasmic Ca^{2+} concentration. Arguments for (4) and against
(5) the calcium mobilization theory have been presented and a
recent review gives some of the background (6).

---

[1]Abbreviations used: PtdIns, phosphatidylinositol; PtdIns
4P, phosphatidylinositol 4-phosphate (diphosphoinositide);
PtdIns 4,5P$_2$, phosphatidylinositol 4,5-bisphosphate (tri-
phosphoinositide).

CALCIUM REGULATION
IN BIOLOGICAL SYSTEMS

117

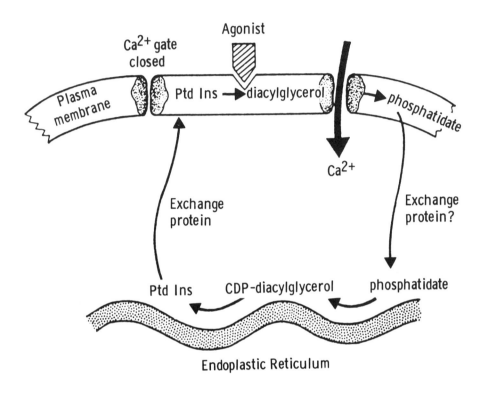

FIGURE 1. Michell's original calcium-gating theory.

$$\text{phosphatidylinositol} + H_2O \longrightarrow \text{diacylglycerol} + \text{inositol 1-phosphate}$$

$$\text{phosphatidylinositol 4-phosphate} + H_2O \longrightarrow \text{diacylglycerol} + \text{inositol 1,4 bisphosphate}$$

$$\text{phosphatidylinositol 4,5 bisphosphate} + H_2O \longrightarrow \text{diacylglycerol} + \text{inositol 1,4,5-triphosphate}$$

FIGURE 2. Catabolism of phosphoinositides by the phospholipase C route.

II. PROBLEMS FOR THE CALCIUM MOBILIZATION THEORY

If receptor-linked phosphoinositide hydrolysis causes the entry or mobilization of Ca^{2+} it should not be dependent upon extracellular Ca^{2+}, a point made quite strongly by Michell (1) in his original formulation of the theory. In more recent versions (7,8) a distinction is made between Ca^{2+} as a "regulatory component" and a requirement for trace quantities of the cation, since as already pointed out, the enzymes hydrolysing phosphoinositides depend upon Ca^{2+}. Whether this distinction is valid or not, a number of tissues do show a phosphoinositide response which is clearly dependent on external Ca^{2+}. In iris muscle, for instance (9) acetylcholine causes increased production of inositol monophosphate and inositol triphosphate, probably because of PtdIns $4,5P_2$ hydrolysis. The acetylcholine effect is Ca^{2+}-dependent and is blocked by calcium antagonists such as verapamil. Influx of Ca^{2+} caused by the ionophore A23187 produces inositol phosphates indistinguishable from those produced in response to acetylcholine. The authors (9) concluded that the phosphoinositide response was secondary to the Ca^{2+}-influx arising from activation of muscarinic receptors.

Cardiac muscarinic receptors stimulate PtdIns turnover and a recent paper (10) shows that PtdIns $4,5P_2$ hydrolysis may occur. The effects are again Ca^{2+}-dependent. The inhibitory (vagal) effects of acetylcholine on the heart are consistent with decreased availability of Ca^{2+}, so once more the results cannot be reconciled with a calcium-mobilizing theory of the phosphoinositide effect.

Muscarinic phosphoinositide responses in brain synaptosomes also require external Ca^{2+}. Measuring only the increased labelling of PtdIns and phosphatidate with $^{32}P_i$, rather than PtdIns $4,5P_2$ breakdown, Griffin et al. (11) found that the muscarinic changes in labelling remained if Ca^{2+} was omitted from the incubation medium. If 0.5 mM EGTA was added to the medium however, the increase in labelling was completely abolished. It was concluded that the relevant receptors were presynaptic, but Agranoff and Fisher (12) conclude from denervation and lesioning studies with guinea pig hippocampus that the muscarinic receptors in that part of the cerebral cortex are post-synaptic. However, the fragment of post-synaptic membrane attached to a synaptosome does not have access to the metabolic mechanisms inside the synaptosome. It seems unlikely therefore that such fragments will display a phosphoinositide response. Agranoff and Fisher's reply to this difficulty is to suggest (12) that the hippocampal synaptosome preparation contains re-sealed dendrite-derived particles or 'dendrosomes', with post-synaptic muscarinic receptors linked to neuronal metabolism. Direct evidence for this is not yet available and it seems clear that presynaptic muscarinic receptors exist in the brain (13), so that the location of the phosphoinositide effect must remain obscure at present. It is also of interest that pharmacological studies suggest the existence of more than one type of muscarinic receptor (13). Whether all types show the same phosphoinositide response is also unknown at this time. Nevertheless, since the response requires external Ca^{2+} it provides no support for a calcium mobilization theory.

Cockroft (14) has listed a number of other tissues in which phosphoinositide changes appear to be caused by calcium mobilization, but it should be remembered that in most of those quoted only PtdIns metabolism was studied. In several, e.g. the platelet, it now seems clear that PtdIns $4,5P_2$ loss is the first lipid response to receptor activation. Space will not allow a detailed account, but Cockroft quotes the following cells or tissues in which the PtdIns response is (a) sensitive to external calcium and (b) triggered by a Ca^{2+} ionophore without the need for receptor activation: neutrophils stimulated by F-met.leu.phe; lymphocytes by phytohaemagglutinin; mast cells by ATP: pancreas by acetylcholine.

In view of these results therefore, it is difficult to uphold the view that phosphoinositides have a universal calcium-mobilizing function.

III. THE ADRENAL MEDULLA

The present paper summarises recent studies in our laboratory and elsewhere on the receptor-linked phosphoinositide metabolism of the adrenal medulla. This tissue was chosen since it presented some unusual features. Earlier work had suggested that muscarinic activation of the bovine medulla increased the labelling of phosphatidylinositol and phosphatidate with [^{32}P]orthophosphate (15,16). However, secretion of catecholamines is a nicotinic response in this species and Fisher et al. (17) showed that there was an accompanying influx of calcium ions which did not occur with purely muscarinic drugs. These workers concluded that the secretory response of the bovine chromaffin cell and the phosphoinositide labelling are separate and distinct processes. We have therefore sought answers to three questions: (a) what is the function of the muscarinic receptors? (b) what is the initial phosphoinositide response to their activation? and (c) is the phosphoinositide response dependent upon calcium ion concentration in the medium?

IV. MUSCARINIC RECEPTORS MODULATE CATECHOLAMINE SECRETION BY PERFUSED ADRENAL MEDULLA

For these experiments, which are reported in more detail elsewhere (18), we used bovine adrenal glands perfused with Locke's solution in a retrograde fashion at 35°. One gland served as a control and the other was perfused with Locke's solution containing 10^{-4} M muscarine or 10^{-4} M pilocarpine as muscarinic agonists. Catecholamine secretion was stimulated by the injection of 4 ml 3 x 10^{-4} M nicotine into the tube carrying perfusion fluid just before it entered the gland. The perfusate was collected in 2 min fractions for the estimation of catecholamines (19).

In glands perfused with Locke's solution containing a muscarinic drug secretion due to nicotine was inhibited by 40%, suggesting that the muscarinic receptor in the bovine adrenal medulla is inhibitory. This is in accord with the results of Derome et al. (20) and Fisher et al. (17). In other species such as the chicken or cat, muscarinic receptor activation will stimulate the secretion of catecholamines (references in 18).

The mechanism of this inhibitory muscarinic action is not understood, though there are claims that muscarinic agents promote efflux of Ca^{2+} from chromaffin cells and also raise the intracellular concentration of cyclic GMP (21).

V. THE INITIAL PHOSPHOINOSITIDE RESPONSE TO MUSCARINIC ACTIVATION

Abdel-Latif et al. (22) showed in 1977 that muscarinic stimuli caused breakdown of phosphatidylinositol 4,5 bisphosphate (PtdIns 4,5P$_2$) rather than PtdIns in the iris muscle. Since then this rapid hydrolysis of PtdIns 4,5P$_2$ has been seen in several types of cells in response to receptors which mobilize calcium. It is probably the first phosphoinositide change caused by receptor activation.

For studies of the muscarinic system of the bovine adrenal medulla, we have used chromaffin cells in culture (17). After 2 days in culture the cells were labelled with [^{32}P]orthophosphate for 75 min and after two washes to remove excess radioactivity the medium was replaced by Locke's solution containing carbachol or muscarine (3 x 10^{-4} M). After 30 sec, trichloroacetic acid was added and lipids were extracted from the resulting precipitate with acidified chloroform-methanol. After separation by one-dimensional thin-layer chromatography (23), the radioactivity of phosphatidic acid and the phosphoinositides was determined for comparison with lipids from control cells incubated without the muscarinic agonists.

In the 30 sec incubation carbachol or muscarine produced a roughly 20% loss of radioactivity from PtdIns $4,5P_2$ and PtdIns 4P, along with a 60% increase of ^{32}P in phosphatidate (Table I). The probable explanation is that the polyphosphoinositides were hydrolysed to inositol phosphates and diacylglycerol and that the latter was phosphorylated to phosphatidate by diacylglycerol kinase. No changes in the labelling of PtdIns were seen during this brief incubation. Our results for the polyphosphoinositides are very similar to those of Creba et al. (2) who worked with pre-labelled hepatocytes. Similar rapid breakdown of PtdIns $4,5P_2$ induced by activation of cell surface receptors has been reported now for platelets (24), synaptosomes from brain (12), rat parotid acinar cells (25) and pancreatic acinar cells (26).

VI. MUSCARINIC BREAKDOWN OF POLYPHOSPHOINOSITIDES REQUIRES EXTERNAL CALCIUM

There is considerable discussion at present about the calcium requirement for the similar rapid hydrolysis of polyphosphoinositides in rat hepatocytes. Creba et al. (2) find a partial requirement for external calcium, Williamson and his colleagues consider the changes to be independent of external calcium (27) but Exton and his group insist on a full requirement (28,29). Our results for the chromaffin cell agree with those of Exton et al. When calcium was omitted from the Locke's solution (usual concentration 2.2 mM) muscarinic drugs were entirely without effect on the polyphosphoinositides (Table I).

VII. DISCUSSION

If polyphosphoinositide breakdown in response to muscarinic receptor activation is somehow mobilizing calcium within the chromaffin cell, it is not easy to understand why external calcium is needed for the breakdown. The same argument applies to vasopressin-induced hydrolysis of PtdIns $4,5P_2$ in hepatocytes. In the chromaffin cell things are even more confusing since muscarinic action does not appear to increase the concentration of Ca^{2+} in the cytoplasm (17) and may in fact cause efflux of this cation (21). However, these experiments measured only movements of ^{45}Ca and more precise measurements

Table I. Rapid Changes in Polyphosphoinositide and Phosphatidate Labelling in Response to Brief Incubation of Adrenal Chromaffin Cells with Carbachol

	Medium Ca^{2+} (mM)	PtdIns $4,5P_2$	PtdIns $4P$	Phosphatidate
Control	2.2	592 ± 190	306 ± 25	202 ± 60
Carbachol	2.2	477 ± 123	231 ± 100	322 ± 20
Carbachol	0	580 ± 144	325 ± 175	288 ± 23
Carbachol	0 (0.5 mM EGTA)	584 ± 146	320 ± 162	261 ± 45

Cells were pre-incubated with [^{32}P]orthophosphate for 60 min and after washing away excess radioactivity they were incubated for 30 sec only with 3 x 10^{-4} M carbachol. Figures represent c.p.m. ± S.D. and are means of 6 experiments. Each incubation tube contained the same volume of cell suspension. Similar results were obtained with the same concentration of muscarine.

of intracellular calcium concentration in the chromaffin cell
are required, possibly using an intracellular calcium indica-
tor (30). At present it can only be said that there is no
support from experiments with bovine chromaffin cells for the
concept that polyphosphoinositide hydrolysis causes mobilization of calcium.

Presynaptic muscarinic receptors have been demonstrated in
the electric tissue of Torpedo marmorata (31), the work being
suggested by the increased labelling of PtdIns which was seen
when the electric organ was stimulated in situ (32). Such
increased turnover seemed likely to be associated with
muscarinic receptors even though the cholinergic system of the
organ was widely held until then to be entirely nicotinic.
These muscarinic receptors inhibit the release of acetylcholine (33,34) in much the same way as the muscarinic receptors
of adrenal medulla inhibit catecholamine release. Michaelson
and colleagues (34) suggest that prostaglandins, in particular
PGE_2, mediate the inhibitory effect of muscarinic agonists in
T. marmorata electric organ. As claimed by Marshall et al.
(35), phospholipase A_2 acting on PtdIns is considered to provide arachidonic acid for PGE_2 synthesis. This is not the
ideal explanation for a phosphoinositide effect however.
Other phospholipids can provide arachidonic acid by this route
and are often better substrates for phospholipase A_2, while
PtdIns is preferentially hydrolysed by the phospholipase C
route in extracts of most tissues studied. If prostaglandin
release is to be the explanation of the phosphoinositide
effect in adrenal medulla, it will be necessary to explain the
observed loss of PtdIns $4,5P_2$. As has been suggested for the
platelet, diacylglycerol rich in arachidonic acid would have
to be released first and the arachidonic then freed by lipase
action. This seems unnecessarily complex, unless there are
regulatory mechanisms of which we are unaware.

As already mentioned, there is now evidence for more than
one type of muscarinic receptor (13). One way out of the difficulties for the calcium mobilization theory which the inhibitory receptors of adrenal medulla and heart (10) present,
would be the finding of some major difference in the
phosphoinositide responses associated with excitatory (calcium
mobilizing) and inhibitory (calcium restricting?) muscarinic
receptors. This does not seem to be the case, however. In
fact our present study of adrenal medulla gives results strik-
ingly similar to those for the hepatocyte, as mentioned above.

A recent paper (36) suggests that the inositol
triphosphate released when PtdIns $4,5P_2$ is hydrolysed acts as
a 'second messenger' mobilizing calcium from intracellular
stores (see also comment in the same journal, reference 27).
Michell and Lapetina (38) claimed in 1972 that inositol
1,2-cyclic phosphate acted in a similar way, but the theory

was short-lived. In many ways inositol 1,4,5-triphosphate is a more attractive candidate, especially since the 1,4-bisphosphate is said to be inactive so that enzymic conversion of the former to the latter would switch off the effect. However, it is not easy to see why the release of the inositol triphosphate in response to surface receptor activation should be dependent on external calcium, if that indeed proves to be the case when the hepatocyte experiments have been repeated. This would also be a problem with the chromaffin cell if PtdIns $4,5P_2$ hydrolysis is releasing 'second messenger' triphosphate. One of the most interesting chemical features of the polyphosphoinositides and one that is probably shared by inositol 1,4,5-triphosphate, is the ability to chelate Ca^{2+} (reviewed in reference 6). This plays no particular part in the second messenger theory. In addition we have no clear idea as yet about the nature of the internal store from which the messenger is said to mobilize Ca^{2+}. If it is surrounded by a membrane, it seems unlikely that the inositol triphosphate could enter. By analogy with c-AMP, it may be that the triphosphate activates a protein kinase, which then causes mobilization of Ca^{2+}.

Another possibility has been suggested elsewhere by one of us (6). There is evidence from more than one tissue that the plasma membrane Ca^{2+}-dependent ATPase responsible for removing Ca^{2+} from the cytoplasm may be activated by PtdIns $4,5P_2$. Activation of receptors which mobilize calcium is known to cause hydrolysis of this lipid, thus reducing the outward flow of this cation and reinforcing the receptor effect (Fig. 3). There is also suggestive evidence (39) that B50 kinase, which is similar to C kinase of Nishizuka (40) inhibits synthesis of PtdIns $4,5P_2$. Thus (Fig. 3) the release of diacylglycerol from this lipid could activate C kinase and prevent resynthesis until the diacylglycerol has been converted to phosphatidate. Whether the activation of the Ca^{2+}-pump ATPase by PtdIns $4,5P_2$ is itself mediated by a kinase is at present unknown.

Work is in progress to study the Ca^{2+}-ATPase and PtdIns $4,5P_2$ further in adrenal medulla. However, the theory outlined here does not get over the difficulties presented by polyphosphoinositide-linked muscarinic receptors which do not seem to mobilize calcium.

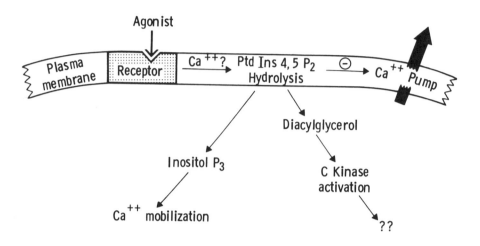

FIGURE 3. PtdIns 4,5P_2 and calcium-mobilizing receptors: some possibilities.

REFERENCES

1. Michell, R. H., Biochim. Biophys. Acta 415:81 (1975).
2. Creba, J. A., Downes, C. P., Hawkins, P. T., Brewster, G., Michell, R. H., and Kirk, C. J., Biochem. J. 212:733 (1983).
3. Kemp, P., Hubscher, G., and Hawthorne, J. N., Biochem. J. 79:193 (1961).
4. Michell, R. H., Nature 296:492 (1982).
5. Hawthorne, J. N., Nature 295:281 (1982).
6. Hawthorne, J. N., Bioscience Reports 3:887 (1983).
7. Michell, R. H., and Kirk, C. J., Trends Pharm. Sci. 2:86 (1981).
8. Michell, R. H., Kirk, C. J., Jones, L. M., Downes, C. P., and Creba, J. A., Phil. Trans. Roy. Soc. Lond. B296:123 (1981).
9. Akhtar, R. A., and Abdel-Latif, A. A., Biochem. J. 192:783 (1980).
10. Brown, S. L., and Brown, J. H., Molec. Pharmacol. 24:351 (1984).
11. Griffin, H. D., Hawthorne, J. N., Sykes, M., and Orlacchio, A., Biochem. Pharmacol. 28:1143 (1979).

12. Agranoff, B. W., and Fisher, S. K., in "Phospholipids in the Nervous System, Vol. 1" (L. A. Horrocks, G. B. Ansell, and G. Procellati, eds.), p. 301. Raven Press, New York, 1982.

13. Caulfield, M., and Straughan, D., Trends Neurosci. 6:73 (1983).

14. Cockroft, S., Trends Pharm. Sci. 2:340 (1981).

15. Hokin, M. R., Benfrey, B. G., and Hokin, L. E., J. Biol. Chem. 233:814 (1958).

16. Trifaro, J. M., Molec. Pharmacol. 5:382 (1969).

17. Fisher, S. K., Holz, R. W., and Agranoff, B. W., J. Neurochem. 37:491 (1981).

18. Swilem, A-M. F., Hawthorne, J. N., and Azila N., Biochem. Pharmacol. 32:3873 (1983).

19. Azila, N., and Hawthorne, J. N., Biochem. J. 204:291 (1982).

20. Derome, G., Tseng, R., Mercier, P., Lemaire, I., and Lemaire, S., Biochem. Pharmacol. 30:855 (1981).

21. Ohsako, S., and Deguchi, T., FEBS Lett. 152:62 (1983).

22. Abdel-Latif, A. A., Akhtar, R. A., and Hawthorne, J. N., Biochem. J. 162:61 (1977).

23. Van Rooijen, L. A. A., Seguin, E. B., and Agranoff, B. W., Biochem. Biophys. Res. Commun. 112:919 (1983).

24. Billah, M. M., and Lapetina, E. G., Biochem. Biophys. Res. Commun. 109:217 (1982).

25. Weiss, S. J., McKinney, J. S., and Putney, J. W. Jr., Molec. Pharm. 23:71 (1983).

26. Putney, J. W. Jr., Burgess, G. M., Halenda, S. P., McKinney, J. S., and Rubin, R. P., Biochem. J. 212:483 (1983).

27. Thomas, A. P., Marks, J. S., Coll, K. E., and Williamson, J. R., J. Biol. Chem. 258:5716 (1983).

28. Prpic, V., Blackmore, P. F., and Exton, J. H., J. Biol. Chem. 257:11323 (1982).

29. Rhodes, D., Prpic, V., Exton, J. H., and Blackmore, P. F., J. Biol. Chem. 258:2770 (1983).

30. Tsien, R. Y., Pozzau, T., and Rink, T. J., J. Cell Biol. 94:325 (1982).

31. Pickard, M. R., and Strange, P. G., Biochem. Soc. Trans. 6:129 (1978).

32. Bleasdale, J. E., Hawthorne, J. N., Widlund, L., and Heilbronn, E., Biochem. J. 158:557 (1976).

33. Dowdall, M. J., Golds, P. R., and Strange, P. G., in "Presynaptic Receptors: Mechanism and Function" (J. De Belleroche, ed.), p. 103. Ellis Horwood, Chichester, 1982.

34. Pinchasi, I., Shanietski, B., Schwartzman, M., Raz, A., and Michaelson, D. M., in "Presynaptic Receptors: Mechanism and Function" (J. De Belleroche, ed.), p. 114.

Ellis Horwood, Chichester, 1982.

35. Marshall, P. J., Boatman, D. E., and Hokin, L. E., J. Biol. Chem. 256:844 (1981).

36. Streb, H., Irvine, R. F., Berridge, M. J., and Schulz, I., Nature, 306:67 (1983).

37. Hesketh, R., Nature, 306:16 (1983).

38. Michell, R. H., and Lapetina, E. G., Nature New Biol. 240:258 (1972).

39. Aloyo, V. J., Zwiess, H., and Gispen, W. H., J. Neurochem. 41:649 (1983).

40. Nishizuka, Y., Phil. Trans. Roy. Soc. Lond. B. 302:101 (1983).

POSSIBLE ROLE OF CALMODULIN-DEPENDENT PROTEIN KINASE IN NERVE FUNCTIONS[1]

Hitoshi Fujisawa
Takashi Yamauchi
Sachiko Okuno
Hiroyasu Nakata

Department of Biochemistry
Asahikawa Medical College
Asahikawa

I. INTRODUCTION

Calcium ion and cyclic AMP are the main components of an internal signaling system which regulates the activity of most cells. Since both intracellular signals are present in almost every cell, the interaction between the regulatory effects of Ca^{2+} and cyclic AMP on cellular processes in a variety of cells is of great importance. Calcium ion has a central role in stimulus-secretion coupling in a number of cells including neuronal cells (1). In this chapter, we would like to discuss our recent studies on the regulation of the function of neuronal cells by Ca^{2+} and cyclic AMP, via calmodulin-dependent protein kinase and cyclic AMP-dependent protein kinase.

The major function of neuronal cells is to synthesize, store and release neurotransmitters such as acetylcholine, serotonin, dopamine, noradrenaline and so on. The neuron is made up of a nerve cell body, its afferent extension (termed

[1]This work has been supported in part by Grants-in-Aid for Scientific Research from the Ministry of Education, Science and Culture of Japan, and by grants from the Naito Research Foundation (1975, 1980), the Byotai Taisha Research Foundation (1976), the Takeda Science Foundation (1979) and the Chiyoda-Seimei Foundation (1980, 1981).

dendrite) and its efferent extension (termed axon). Since the axon has no apparent protein-synthesizing capability, the enzymes involved in the synthesis of neurotransmitters are synthesized in nerve cell bodies and are transported down the axon to the axonal terminal where they are put to work. The neurotransmitters which are synthesized in the axonal terminal are stored in synaptic vesicles. In response to a nerve stimulus, the neurotransmitter is released by fusion of the vesicles to the plasma membrane. Vesicle fusion is known to be triggered by Ca^{2+} influx, and recent studies have strongly suggested that calmodulin mediates Ca^{2+} action in exocytosis at the nerve terminal (2), although the molecular mechanism is still only poorly understood. In spite of marked fluctuations in the neuronal activities, the levels of neurotransmitters within the nerve terminals remain relatively constant. Thus, an efficient regulatory mechanism must operate to modulate the rate of synthesis of neurotransmitters, depending on need. Most of the regulatory effects must be exerted by regulation of the activity of tyrosine 3-monooxygenase, because this is the rate-limiting enzyme in the biosynthesis of catecholamines (3,4).

II. CALMODULIN-DEPENDENT PROTEIN KINASE II IN RAT BRAIN

In 1980 we demonstrated the existence of three distinct calmodulin-dependent protein kinases in rat brain cytosol and these were termed calmodulin-dependent protein kinase I, II, and III on the basis of their order of elution from a column of Sepharose CL-6B (5). Calmodulin-dependent protein kinase I with an apparent molecular weight of about one million showed the phosphorylase kinase activity which is stimulated by the addition of calmodulin in the presence of Ca^{2+}. Therefore, it may be identical to phosphorylase kinase (6,7). Calmodulin-dependent protein kinase II with an apparent molecular weight of about 500,000 is the new calmodulin-dependent protein kinase which is involved in the activation of tryptophan 5-monooxygenase. Tryptophan 5-monooxygenase is the rate-limiting enzyme in the biosynthesis of serotonin in the nervous system (8,9). This kinase phosphorylates not only tryptophan 5-monooxygenase but also casein and myosin light chain. Calmodulin-dependent protein kinase III with an apparent molecular weight of about 100,000 resembles myosin light chain kinase (10), since it shows a relatively high activity of myosin light chain kinase. Although calmodulin-dependent protein kinase III phosphorylates casein also, myosin light chain kinase from muscle (11) or platelet (12) cannot use it as a substrate.

Thus, there are three distinct calmodulin-dependent protein kinases which differ from each other in molecular size
and substrate specificity. One is a so-called phosphorylase
kinase, another is a so-called myosin light chain kinase, and
the third is the new enzyme, termed calmodulin-dependent protein kinase II. This enzyme was purified to apparent homogeneity and its properties were extensively studied in our
laboratory (13).

The molecular weight of calmodulin-dependent protein
kinase II as determined by the sedimentation equilibrium
method is about 540,000. The molecular weight as determined
by sodium dodecyl sulfate-polyacrylamide gel electrophoresis
is 55,000. These results indicate that calmodulin-dependent
protein kinase II is composed of about ten probably identical
subunits. The kinetic properties as determined by measuring
the activation of tryptophan 5-monooxygenase are as follows:
K_m for ATP is about 60 μM, K_a for calmodulin is 10 nM and K_a
for Ca^{2+} is 1.6 μM.

Similar calmodulin-dependent protein kinases have recently
been independently reported in rat brain from DeLorenzo's
laboratory (14) and from Miyamoto's laboratory (15).
DeLorenzo's Ca^{2+}-calmodulin tubulin kinase has been reported
to have a major calmodulin-binding peptide with a molecular
weight of 55,000. Miyamoto's calmodulin-dependent protein
kinase has been well characterized and its properties are very
similar to those of calmodulin-dependent protein kinase II.
These results together with others suggest that these three
enzymes may be identical (16). More recently, it has been
demonstrated that synapsin I kinase II reported by Kennedy and
Greengard (17) in rat brain exhibits a major protein staining
band with a molecular weight of about 50,000 on sodium dodecyl
sulfate-polyacrylamide gel electrophoresis, and a monoclonal
antibody prepared against synapsin I kinase II cross-reacts
with glycogen synthase kinase from skeletal muscle (18).
These results suggest the possibility that calmodulin-
dependent protein kinase II reported from our laboratory,
Ca^{2+}-calmodulin tubulin kinase from DeLorenzo's laboratory,
calmodulin-dependent protein kinase from Miyamoto's laboratory, and synapsin I kinase II from Greengard's laboratory are
all the same enzyme and may be closely related to calmodulin-
dependent glycogen synthase kinase.

A prominent feature of calmodulin-dependent protein kinase
II is that this enzyme occurs in highest abundance in neuronal
tissues such as cerebral cortex, brainstem and cerebellum
(19), while the so-called phosphorylase kinase and myosin
light chain kinase are widely distributed in a variety of
tissues. Other tissues tested, including adrenal gland, lung,
kidney, testis, spleen, skeletal muscle, liver and heart
showed little, if any, activity of calmodulin-dependent pro-

tein kinase II (19). When rat brain is fractionated according to the method of Whittaker and Barker (20) and subcellular distribution of calmodulin-dependent protein kinase II is examined, this kinase appears to occur in the cytosol of both cell bodies and nerve terminals (21).

Another striking feature of calmodulin-dependent protein kinase II is its broad substrate specificity. When the phosphorylation of proteins is examined by autoradiographical analysis, calmodulin-dependent protein kinase II phosphorylates qualitatively and quantitatively many more endogenous proteins than the other two calmodulin-dependent protein kinases (5), indicating it may play a number of roles in the functioning of the central nervous system. The proteins which have so far been identified as substrates of calmodulin-dependent protein kinase II in our laboratory are tryptophan 5-monooxygenase, tyrosine 3-monooxygenase, tubulin, microtubule-associated protein 2 (MAP 2), casein and myosin light chain (22). The K_m values of the enzyme for tryptophan 5-monooxygenase, tubulin, MAP 2, casein and myosin light chain are 0.0003, 1.7, 0.2, 20, and 50 μM, respectively. It should be noted that the K_m values for endogenous protein substrates such as tryptophan 5-monooxygenase, tubulin and MAP 2 are much lower than those for casein and myosin light chain. It should also be noted that the apparent K_m values of calmodulin-dependent protein kinase II for the endogenous protein substrates are considerably lower than their average molar concentrations in brain tissues. The average concentrations of tryptophan 5-monooxygenase in rat brainstem, tyrosine 3-monooxygenase in rat striatum, tubulin in rat brain and MAP 2 in rat brain are roughly estimated to be 0.025, 0.15, 25, and 0.5 μM, respectively (22). These results suggest that these four proteins may be physiological substrates of calmodulin-dependent protein kinase II. It is of particular interest that calmodulin-dependent protein kinase II is particularly abundant in the nervous tissues and these four protein substrates also occur either exclusively or in highest abundance in the nervous tissues.

Myelin basic protein, which has been reported to be a protein substrate of the calmodulin-dependent protein kinase reported by Miyamoto and his co-workers (15), may be a substrate of calmodulin-dependent protein kinase II.

III. REGULATION OF TYROSINE 3-MONOOXYGENASE ACTIVITY

Calmodulin-dependent protein kinase II is involved in the activation of not only tryptophan 5-monooxygenase but also tyrosine 3-monooxygenase. Although both tryptophan

5-monooxygenase (23) and tyrosine 3-monooxygenase (24) were purified to apparent homogeneity from rat sources and their properties extensively studied, no highly reactive antibody to tryptophan 5-monooxygenase has been available. Therefore, the relationship between phosphorylation and activation of the enzyme by calmodulin-dependent protein kinase II was examined with tyrosine 3-monooxygenase. The incorporation of phosphate into tyrosine 3-monooxygenase by calmodulin-dependent protein kinase II was demonstrated by immunoprecipitation followed by sodium dodecyl sulfate-polyacrylamide gel electrophoresis. When the activation of tyrosine 3-monooxygenase is examined using purified calmodulin-dependent protein kinase II, it requires the third protein, called activator protein, as well as calmodulin and calmodulin-dependent protein kinase II (25). In contrast to activation, phosphorylation of the monooxygenase requires calmodulin-dependent protein kinase II and calmodulin but does not require the presence of activator protein. Thus, activation and phosphorylation of the monooxygenase by calmodulin-dependent protein kinase II are distinct reactions, and phosphorylation of the monooxygenase by calmodulin-dependent protein kinase II appears to be necessary for the activation by activator protein. In other words, the activation of the monooxygenase by calmodulin-dependent protein kinase II may occur in two steps. The first step is the phosphorylation of the enzyme by calmodulin-dependent protein kinase II and the second is the activation of the phosphory-lated enzyme by activator protein.

Activator protein is composed of two identical subunits, the molecular weight of which is 35,000 (25). The fact that the activator protein was purified to homogeneity by a purifi-cation of only 130-fold from rat brain cytosol indicates its very high content in brain tissues. The activity of the acti-vator protein was widely distributed in all of the tissues tested, such as cerebral cortex, brainstem, adrenal gland, liver, heart and skeletal muscle, although the highest specif-ic activity was observed in brain tissues, indicating that activator protein may play its role not only in the regulation of monoamine biosynthesis but also in other physiological functions in various tissues.

Tyrosine 3-monooxygenase is activated also by cyclic AMP-dependent protein kinase (26), although tryptophan 5-monooxygenase is not. When the pH profile for the tyrosine 3-monooxygenase activity of the extract from rat striatum, where tyrosine 3-monooxygenase exists most abundantly, was examined, it showed a sharp pH optimum with maximum activity occurring at pH 5.4 and very little, if any, activity at or above pH 7. When the extract was incubated at 30°C for 1 hour with dibutyryl-cyclic AMP in the presence of Mg^{2+} and the ATP-generating system, the tyrosine 3-monooxygenase activity showed a broad pH optimum over the pH range of 5.5 - 7.5. It is worth noting that the activation magnitude is one hundred times or more at pH 7.0, since the intracellular pH has been reported to be 7.0 - 7.1 (27,28).

In contrast, when the rat brain extract was incubated with Ca^{2+} at 30°C for 1 hour under the phosphorylating conditions, the tyrosine 3-monooxygenase activity showed a pH profile similar to that of the original non-phosphorylated enzyme, although it was activated about twice over the pH range of 5.5 to 8.0. Thus, the extent of the activation of tyrosine 3-monooxygenase by calmodulin-dependent protein kinase II is much smaller at a physiological pH (pH 7) than that by cyclic AMP-dependent protein kinase.

In order to understand the relationship between the activation of tyrosine 3-monooxygenase by cyclic AMP-dependent protein kinase and the activation by calmodulin-dependent protein kinase II and activator protein, the extract from rat striatum was incubated with Ca^{2+} and dibutyryl cyclic AMP together under the phosphorylating conditions. When assayed at pH 7.0, the enzyme is activated about one hundred fold by incubation with dibutyryl cyclic AMP and this activation is further stimulated in the presence of Ca^{2+}, whereas the stimulative effect of Ca^{2+} is relatively small in the absence of cyclic AMP. Thus, the activation of the enzyme by both cyclic AMP-dependent protein kinase and calmodulin-dependent protein kinase II together is greater than an additive activation. The results described above, taken together, suggest that the activity of tyrosine 3-monooxygenase may be regulated by both cyclic AMP and Ca^{2+} <u>via</u> cyclic AMP-dependent protein kinase and calmodulin-dependent protein kinase II, respectively, in the nervous system, and further suggest that the primary regulator may be cyclic AMP with Ca^{2+} helping its action.

IV. REGULATION OF MICROTUBULE ASSEMBLY-DISASSEMBLY

Microtubule proteins such as tubulin and MAP 2 are also good substrates of calmodulin-dependent protein kinase II, as described above. On the other hand, cyclic AMP-dependent protein kinase has also been demonstrated to catalyze phosphorylation of MAP 2 (29,30). The apparent K_m value of calmodulin-dependent protein kinase II for MAP 2 is about 0.2 μM, which is one order of magnitude lower than that of cyclic AMP-dependent protein kinase (31). In order to understand the physiological significance of phosphorylation of microtubule proteins by calmodulin-dependent protein kinase II and cyclic AMP-dependent protein kinase, the effects of the phosphorylation on microtubule assembly were examined. Microtubule assembly and disassembly can be monitored spectrophotometrically by measuring the turbidity at 350 nm. When calmodulin-dependent protein kinase II or cyclic AMP-dependent protein kinase is added under phosphorylating conditions to the microtubules assembled by incubation with GTP at 37°C, microtubule disassembly occurs even at that temperature. The initial velocity of this disassembly is much faster in the presence of excess calmodulin-dependent protein kinase II than in the presence of excess cyclic AMP-dependent protein kinase. Thus, calmodulin-dependent protein kinase II and cyclic AMP-dependent protein kinase are both involved in controlling the assembly and disassembly of microtubules in a similar manner, but the former is more effective. This indicates that the primary regulator in controlling the assembly and disassembly of microtubules may be Ca^{2+} and that cyclic AMP may help its action.

These findings suggest that calmodulin-dependent protein kinase II is involved not only in the regulation of the biosynthesis of monoamine neurotransmitters, but also in the regulation of dynamic cellular processes such as neurotransmitter secretion in the nervous system, since microtubule proteins are known to occur abundantly in the brain tissues and to function in dynamic cellular processes such as cell secretion and intracellular transport (32).

It will be of importance to know which is involved in controlling microtubule assembly-disassembly, phosphorylation of tubulin or phosphorylation of MAP 2. In order to resolve this, tubulin and MAP 2 were purified to apparent homogeneity on sodium dodecyl sulfate-polyacrylamide gel electrophoresis from rat brain and the relationship between the phosphorylation of each protein and microtubule assembly was examined. When the purified MAP 2 is incubated with the purified tubulin at 37°C in the presence of GTP and Mg^{2+}, absorbance at 350 nm is increased. A similar increase in the absorbancy is also observed when MAP 2 is incubated with the tubulin which has been phosphorylated by calmodulin-dependent protein kinase II. On the other hand, when the MAP 2 previously phosphorylated by calmodulin-dependent protein kinase II is used in place of non-phosphorylated MAP 2 in these experiments, such a remarkable increase in the absorbance at 350 nm is not observed. These results indicate that phosphorylation of MAP 2 is involved in the regulation of microtubule assembly-disassembly but phosphorylation of tubulin is not. Burke and DeLorenzo (33,34) have also discussed the possibility that Ca^{2+}-stimulated phosphorylation of tubulin is not directly involved in microtubule formation. Thus, calmodulin-dependent protein kinase II appears to be involved in controlling microtubule assembly-disassembly via phosphorylation of MAP 2. Phosphorylation of tubulin by calmodulin-dependent protein

kinase II may be involved in the regulation of some other
functions of microtubules in the nervous system.

V. POSSIBLE REGULATORY ROLE OF Ca^{2+} AND C-AMP
IN NERVE FUNCTIONS

The major function of the neuronal cell is secretion of
neurotransmitters followed by their synthesis. Based on the
results so far described, a possible mechanism for the regulation of neuronal cell function by calmodulin-dependent protein
kinase II and cyclic AMP-dependent protein kinase is presented
in Fig. 1. In response to a stimulus, the axonal terminal is
initiated to depolarize and its depolarization results in an
influx of Ca^{2+} into the axonal terminal. As a result, Ca^{2+}
binds to calmodulin and consequently activates calmodulin-
dependent protein kinase II which phosphorylates a variety of

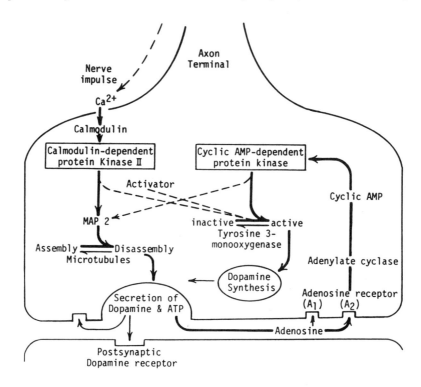

FIGURE 1. A possible mechanism for the regulation of
nerve cell function by calmodulin-dependent protein kinase II
and cyclic AMP-dependent protein kinase in the dopaminergic
neuron.

endogenous proteins including microtubule proteins, such as MAP 2 and tubulin, and tyrosine 3-monooxygenase in the case of catecholaminergic neurons such as dopaminergic neuron. Phosphorylation of MAP 2 induces disassembly of microtubules. Since it has been believed that microtubule assembly-disassembly is related to dynamic cellular processes such as intracellular transport and cell secretion and that the release of neurotransmitters from nerve terminals occurs as a result of an increase in the intracellular level of Ca^{2+} (1), it is conceivable that phosphorylation of MAP 2 by calmodulin-dependent protein kinase II promotes the release of a neurotransmitter such as dopamine, probably by a process of exocytosis. On the other hand, cyclic AMP-dependent protein kinase also phosphorylates MAP 2, resulting in disassembly of microtubules. Thus, calmodulin-dependent protein kinase II and cyclic AMP-dependent protein kinase are both involved in controlling microtubule assembly-disassembly in a similar manner, but calmodulin-dependent protein kinase II is more effective. This indicates that the primary regulator in controlling the assembly-disassembly of microtubules involved in dynamic cellular processes such as cell secretion may be Ca^{2+}, and that cyclic AMP may help its action. Immunocytochemical studies have demonstrated that MAP 2 occurs only in neuronal cells (35,36) and is present in dendrites (36,37). Further investigations will be necessary to decide whether MAP 2 exists in axons and nerve terminals.

The current view is that the storage vesicles contain ATP and that it is released from the nerve terminal along with catecholamine on nerve transmission. There is considerable evidence suggesting that adenosine functions as a neuromodulator, probably via presynaptic membrane-localized extracellular receptors (38), sometimes referred to as "adenosine receptors." Two distinct adenosine receptors appear to exist, A_1 receptor which responds to lower concentrations of adenosine and consequently brings about a decrease in cyclic AMP level and A_2 receptor which responds to higher concentrations of adenosine, causing an increase in the level of cyclic AMP (39-41). Perlman and his co-workers (42) have demonstrated that an adenosine derivative promotes the accumulation of cyclic AMP and increases the activity of tyrosine 3-monooxygenase in intact rat pheochromocytoma cells.

In accordance with the current view described above, the following speculation can be made: the ATP released simultaneously with a neurotransmitter on depolarization of the nerve terminal is rapidly degraded to adenosine, which promotes the accumulation of cyclic AMP in the cell via adenosine receptors. The rise in cyclic AMP in the cell activates cyclic AMP-dependent protein kinase, which catalyzes the conversion of tyrosine-3-monooxygenase from inactive form to active form.

The activation of tyrosine 3-monooxygenase is further enhanced by the coordinated action of calmodulin-dependent protein kinase II and activator protein. Thus, cyclic AMP may be the primary regulator controlling the activity of tyrosine 3-monooxygenase and Ca^{2+} appears to help its action. On the other hand, it has been shown that adenosine reduces calcium potentials and depresses the release of neurotransmitters by interfering with depolarization-induced Ca^{2+} fluxes (38). A fall in intracellular Ca^{2+} level halts the action of calmodulin-dependent protein kinase II, leading to depression of the release of neurotransmitters. Depression of the release of neurotransmitters and ATP results in a decrease of cyclic AMP concentration in the cell, which in turn halts the action of cyclic AMP-dependent protein kinase. Consequently, tyrosine 3-monooxygenase is converted from active form to the original inactive form.

In summary, our tentative scheme suggests that the neuronal function in catecholaminergic neurons is regulated by coordinate and sequential effects of the two second messengers, Ca^{2+} and cyclic AMP, via calmodulin-dependent protein kinase II and cyclic AMP-dependent protein kinase. Calcium ion which enters the presynaptic terminal during membrane depolarization is the first signal and cyclic AMP which increases in response to the feedback mechanism probably mediated by adenosine receptors is the second. Although Ca^{2+} and cyclic AMP function in concert to control the secretion and synthesis of catecholamines, Ca^{2+} is more important in stimulating the secretion and cyclic AMP is more important in stimulating the synthesis.

REFERENCES

1. Rubin, R. P., Pharmacol. Rev. 22:389 (1970).
2. Reichardt, L. F., and Kelly, R. B., Ann. Rev. Biochem. 52:871 (1983).
3. Nagatsu, T., Levitt, M., and Udenfriend, S., J. Biol. Chem. 239:2910 (1964).
4. Levitt, M., Spector, S., Sjoerdsma, A., and Udenfriend, S., J. Pharmacol. Exp. Ther. 148:1 (1965).
5. Yamauchi, T., and Fujisawa, H., FEBS Lett. 116:141 (1980).
6. Drummond, G. I., and Bellward, G., J. Neurochem. 17:475 (1970).
7. Ozawa, E., J. Neurochem. 20:1487 (1973).
8. Grahame-Smith, D. G., Biochem. Biophys. Res. Commun. 16:586 (1964).

9. Jéquier, E., Lovenberg, W., and Sjoerdsma, A., Mol.
    Pharmacol. 3:274 (1967).
10. Dabrowska, R., and Hartshorne, D. J., Biochem. Biophys.
    Res. Commun. 85:1352 (1978).
11. Walsh, M. P., Vallet, B., Autric, F., and Demaille, J.
    G., J. Biol. Chem. 254:12136 (1979).
12. Hathaway, D. R., and Adelstein, R. S., Proc. Natl. Acad.
    Sci. USA 76:1653 (1979).
13. Yamauchi, T., and Fujisawa, H., Eur. J. Biochem. 132:15
    (1983).
14. Goldenring, J. R., Gonzalez, B., and DeLorenzo, R. J.,
    Biochem. Biophys. Res. Commun. 108:421 (1982).
15. Fukunaga, K., Yamamoto, H., Matsui, K., Higashi, K., and
    Miyamoto, E., J. Neurochem. 39:1607 (1982).
16. Fujisawa, H., Yamauchi, T., Nakata, H., and Okuno, S., in
    "Calcium and Cell Function, Vol. V" (W. Y. Cheung, ed.),
    in press, Academic Press, New York.
17. Kennedy, M. B., and Greengard, P., Proc. Natl. Acad. Sci.
    USA 78:1293 (1981).
18. McGuinness, T. L., Lai, Y., Greengard, P., Woodgett, J.
    R., and Cohen, P., FEBS Lett. in press.
19. Yamauchi, T., and Fujisawa, H., FEBS Lett. 129:117
    (1981).
20. Whittaker, V. P., and Barker, L. A., Methods of
    Neurochemistry 2:1 (1972).
21. Okuno, S., Yamauchi, T., Nakata, H., and Fujisawa, H.,
    Biogenic Amines, in press.
22. Fujisawa, H., Yamauchi, T., Nakata, H., and Okuno, S., in
    "Molecular Aspects of Cellular Regulation, Vol. 3" (P.
    Cohen, ed.), p. 167. Elsevier/North-Holland and
    Biomedical Press, Amsterdam, 1984.
23. Nakata, H., and Fujisawa, H., Eur. J. Biochem. 122:41
    (1982).
24. Okuno, S., and Fujisawa, H., Eur. J. Biochem. 122:49
    (1982).
25. Yamauchi, T., Nakata, H., and Fujisawa, H., J. Biol.
    Chem. 256:5404 (1981).
26. Fujisawa, H., Yamauchi, T., Nakata, H., and Okuno, S., in
    "Oxygenases and Oxygen Metabolism" (M. Nozaki, S.
    Yamamoto, Y. Ishimura, M. J. Coon, L. Ernster, and R. W.
    Estabrook, eds.), p. 281. Academic Press, New York, 1982.
27. Kjalquist, A., Nardini, M., and Siesjö, B. K., Acta
    Physiol. Scand. 76:485 (1969).
28. Roos, A., Am. J. Physiol. 221:176 (1971).
29. Sloboda, R. D., Rudolph, S. A., Rosenbaum, J. L., and
    Greengard, P., Proc. Natl. Acad. Sci. USA 72:177
    (1975).
30. Rappaport, L., Leterrier, J. F., Virion, A., and Nunez,
    J., Eur. J. Biochem. 62:539 (1976).

31. Theurkauf, W. E., and Vallee, R. B., J. Biol. Chem. 257:3284 (1982).
32. Olmsted, J. B., and Borisy, G. G., Ann. Rev. Biochem. 42:507 (1973).
33. Burke, B. E., and DeLorenzo, R. J., Proc. Natl. Acad. Sci. USA 78:991 (1981).
34. Burke, B. E., and DeLorenzo, R. J., Brain Res. 236:393 (1982).
35. Izant, J. G., and McIntosh, J. R., Proc. Natl. Acad. Sci. USA 77:4741 (1980).
36. Matus, A., Bernhardt, R., and Hugh-Jones, T., Proc. Natl. Acad. Sci. USA 78:3010 (1981).
37. Caceres, A., Payne, M. R., Binder, L. I., and Steward, O., Proc. Natl. Acad. Sci. USA 80:1738 (1983).
38. Lynch, G., and Schubert, P., Ann. Rev. Neurosci. 3:1 (1980).
39. Calker, D. V., Müller, M., and Hamprecht, B., J. Neurochem. 33:999 (1979).
40. Londos, C., Cooper, D. M. F., and Wolff, J., Proc. Natl. Acad. Sci. USA 77:2551 (1980).
41. Bruns, R. F., Can. J. Physiol. Pharmacol. 58:673 (1980).
42. Erny, R. E., Berezo, M. W., and Perlman, R. L., J. Biol. Chem. 256:1335 (1981).

MECHANISMS INVOLVED IN THE ACTIONS
OF CALCIUM DEPENDENT HORMONES ON LIVER

John H. Exton

Howard Hughes Medical Institute and Department of Physiology
Vanderbilt University School of Medicine
Nashville, Tennessee

I. INTRODUCTION

There is now much evidence that the actions of many hormones, neurotransmitters and regulatory agents involve calcium. Examples include the effects of catecholamines, acetylcholine, histamine, oxytocin and prostaglandins on the contraction of certain smooth muscles, of acetylcholine and catecholamines on salivary or lacrimal secretion, of vasopressin and catecholamines on hepatic glycogenolysis, of thrombin and platelet activating factor on platelet activation, of cholecystokinin and acetylcholine on pancreatic acinar secretion, and of the releasing hormones for gonadotrophin and thyrotrophin on the pituitary. A role for calcium in the actions of these and other agents is supported by one or more of the following observations: 1) their actions are impaired in calcium-deficient media, 2) their effects are mimicked by agents which increase intracellular Ca^{2+}, 3) they alter cell or tissue Ca^{2+} fluxes, and 4) they increase cytosolic Ca^{2+}.

The mechanisms by which calcium-dependent hormones and related agents alter cell Ca^{2+} fluxes and raise cytosolic Ca^{2+} have been studied in liver, smooth muscle, salivary gland, platelets and pituitary. The two mechanisms for increasing cytosolic Ca^{2+} are 1) a mobilization of Ca^{2+} from intracellular Ca^{2+} pools such as those in the mitochondria or endoplasmic reticulum or those associated with the plasma membrane or other intracellular membranes, and 2) an alteration in plasma membrane Ca^{2+} permeability and/or $(Ca^{2+}-Mg^{2+})ATPase$ (Ca^{2+} pump) activity such that there is a net influx of extracellular Ca^{2+} (or inhibited efflux of intracellular Ca^{2+}). Mobilization of intracellular Ca^{2+} is usually the initial response to Ca^{2+}-dependent hormones.

Although it is generally agreed that the actions of the calcium-dependent hormones are the result of a rise in cytosolic Ca^{2+}, the primary intracellular targets of cytosolic Ca^{2+} are not fully known. Phosphorylase b kinase, myosin light chain kinase, calmodulin-dependent protein (glycogen synthase) kinase, some membrane (Ca^{2+}-Mg^{2+})ATPases, and troponin C are clearly involved in some tissues, but the enzymes or proteins mediating other responses remain to be identified.

II. CHANGES IN CYTOSOLIC Ca^{2+} INDUCED BY CALCIUM-DEPENDENT HORMONES

There is abundant evidence that epinephrine and norepinephrine acting through the α_1-adrenergic receptor, and also vasopressin and angiotensin II affect Ca^{2+} fluxes in many tissues (for references, see 1). However, the demonstration that these calcium-dependent hormones increase cytosolic Ca^{2+} has been accomplished in only a few instances. Murphy et al. (2) first presented indirect evidence that the α-adrenergic agonist phenylephrine increased cytosolic Ca^{2+} in isolated rat hepatocytes. They employed a method in which the extracellular Ca^{2+} concentration was varied until it was equal to that in the cytosol as shown by the fact that there was no change upon disruption of the cells with digitonin. They calculated that the basal cytosolic Ca^{2+} was 0.2 μM and that the increase with α-adrenergic stimulation was 2- to 3-fold at 2 min. The increase in Ca^{2+} preceded the activation of phosphorylase, and a very good correlation was observed between the dose responses for cytosolic Ca^{2+} and phosphorylase activation.

More recently, Charest et al. (3,4) have used the acetoxymethyl ester of Quin-2, a fluorescent Ca^{2+} chelator (5,6), to measure cytosolic Ca^{2+} in rat hepatocytes. Being uncharged, the ester can enter cells where intracellular esterases release the free compound. This accumulates in the cytosol, but does not penetrate intracellular organelles. When irradiated at 340 nm, the free compound emits fluorescence at 500 nm and this is enhanced 5-fold by Ca^{2+}. Thus the changes in fluorescence in Quin-2-loaded cells can be used to measure cytosolic Ca^{2+}, although corrections may need to be made for changes in basal fluorescence due to alterations in the reduction state of pyridine nucleotides (3).

Figure 1 from Charest et al. (3) shows the increases in cytosolic Ca^{2+} monitored in Quin 2-loaded hepatocytes incubated with epinephrine, phenylephrine, vasopressin and glucagon. The two α-adrenergic agonists increase cytosolic Ca^{2+}

within 2 s and vasopressin produces a similar change after a slight lag. In contrast, the rise in Ca^{2+} with glucagon (10^{-8} M) is slower and has a longer lag. With more physiological concentrations of glucagon (10^{-10} M – 10^{-9} M) the response is delayed and of smaller magnitude. The increase in Ca^{2+} does not appear to play a role in the physiological actions of this hormone (7).

The rise in cytosolic Ca^{2+} induced by maximally effective concentrations of α-adrenergic agonists or vasopressin is from approximately 0.2 μM to 0.6 μM, and precedes the rise in

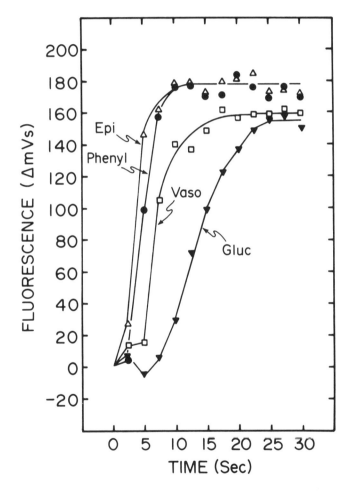

FIGURE 1.   Time courses of fluorescence changes in Quin-2-loaded hepatocytes upon addition of epinephrine (Epi), phenylephrine (Phenyl), vasopressin (Vaso) or glucagon (Gluc). From Charest et al. (3).

phosphorylase $\underline{a}$ (3,4). There is also a very close correlation between the concentration-dependence curves of epinephrine, vasopressin or phenylephrine on cytosolic Ca^{2+} and phosphorylase $\underline{a}$ (3,4). These findings are consistent with Ca^{2+} stimulation of phosphorylase $\underline{b}$ kinase which phosphorylates phosphorylase $\underline{b}$ converting it to phosphorylase $\underline{a}$.

III. MOBILIZATION OF INTRACELLULAR Ca^{2+}
BY CALCIUM-DEPENDENT HORMONES

There is much evidence that Ca^{2+}-dependent hormones initially raise cytosolic Ca^{2+} mainly by mobilizing intracellular Ca^{2+} stores. These hormones cause a rapid large decrease in total cell calcium in hepatocytes (8) or a large release of Ca^{2+} from the perfused liver (9). Since the decrease in cell calcium is much larger than the pool of cytosolic Ca^{2+}, it can be concluded that Ca^{2+} must have been mobilized from intracellular stores (8). More evidence for intracellular Ca^{2+} mobilization comes from the demonstration that the ability of the hormones to activate phosphorylase (10) and to increase cytosolic Ca^{2+} (4) is undiminished on a short-term basis (up to 1 min) when the extracellular Ca^{2+} concentration is decreased by EGTA to such a low concentration that influx of Ca^{2+} into the hepatocytes is abolished. On the other hand, if the reduction in extracellular Ca^{2+} is prolonged, it gradually leads to the depletion of intracellular Ca^{2+} stores with resulting attenuation and loss of all responses (8).

Further support for a major role for intracellular Ca^{2+} mobilization comes from measurements of changes in the calcium content of intracellular organelles. Several studies using atomic absorption spectrometry and other methods have shown that Ca^{2+}-dependent hormones cause a marked reduction in mitochondrial calcium (2,9,11-15) and most workers agree that from a quantitative viewpoint these organelles are a major source of mobilized Ca^{2+}.

Figure 2 shows the dose-response curves for the effects of epinephrine on mitochondrial calcium, phosphorylase $\underline{a}$ and total cell calcium in hepatocytes. The mitochondrial change is elicited by concentrations of the agonist which activate phosphorylase and mobilize total cell calcium. The overall time course of the changes is also consistent with the mitochondria being a major source of mobilized Ca^{2+} (9).

Due to methodological problems, it has not been possible to detect changes in mitochondrial calcium earlier than 30 s after addition of Ca^{2+}-dependent hormones. Thus the possibility must be entertained that these organelles may not be the immediate source of Ca^{2+} mobilized by these hormones.

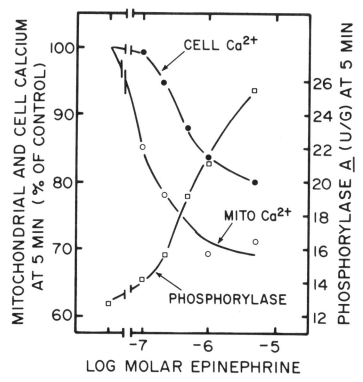

FIGURE 2.   Dose response curves for the effects of epinephrine on phosphorylase a, total cell Ca^{2+} and mitochondrial
Ca^{2+} in hepatocytes. Unpublished data of P. F. Blackmore and
J. -P. Dehaye.

Several groups have suggested that the plasma membrane may be
the initial source of Ca^{2+} (16,17), but efforts to demonstrate
consistent changes in plasma membrane calcium have not been
successful (18).   It has also not been possible to observe
consistent alterations in microsomal calcium.   However,
possible effects on plasma membranes or microsomes might have
been lost during the lengthy isolation procedures for these
fractions.

IV. ALTERATION OF PLASMA MEMBRANE Ca^{2+} FLUXES
BY CALCIUM-DEPENDENT HORMONES

Since intracellular Ca^{2+} stores are of limited magnitude,
any hormone effects based solely on their mobilization will be
of limited duration.   Thus additional hormone effects at the

plasma membrane to alter the efflux or influx of Ca^{2+} would seem necessary to sustain an elevated cytosolic Ca^{2+} concentration and thereby prolong the actions of the Ca^{2+}-dependent hormones.

Studies with the perfused rat liver or isolated hepatocytes have reproducibly shown a large <u>net</u> efflux of Ca^{2+} during the <u>initial</u> stages of epinephrine or vasopressin action (8,19). The efflux of Ca^{2+} is rapid, large but transient. It lasts approximately 5 min and is followed by no detectable net change in medium Ca^{2+} until the hormone is removed or degraded (19). Termination of hormone action is followed by Ca^{2+} uptake to restore the liver calcium content to normal (10,19). Analogous experiments have been carried out with isolated hepatocytes. In cells incubated in media containing physiological levels of Ca^{2+}, vasopressin induces a prolonged rise in cytosolic Ca^{2+} and activation of phosphorylase (4). However, in low Ca^{2+} media (30 μM or less), the

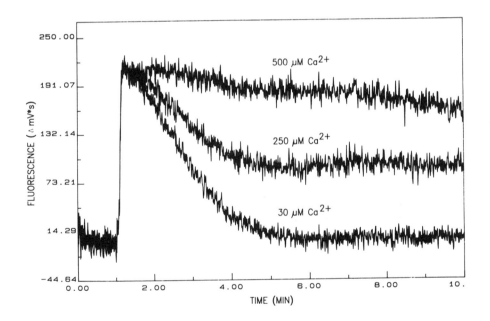

FIGURE 3. Effect of various extracellular Ca^{2+} concentrations on the increase in cytosolic Ca^{2+} induced by vasopressin. Control and Quin-2-loaded hepatocytes were suspended in medium containing 0.5 mM, 0.25 mM or 30 M Ca^{2+} for 5 min before fluorescence measurements were made. The traces shown are the differences between Quin-2 and control fluorescence changes. Vasopressin (10^{-8} μM) was added at 1 min. From Charest <u>et al</u>. (4).

cytosolic Ca^{2+} rise and phosphorylase activation induced by the hormone both decline after about 1 min (Fig. 3), and a second dose of hormone is ineffective (4 and unpublished observations). Readdition of Ca^{2+} to the media restores the hormone responses to an extent dependent upon the concentration of added Ca^{2+} (Fig. 3).

These data illustrate that the magnitude of the hormone effects is influenced by the extracellular Ca^{2+} concentration which can control the level of cytosolic Ca^{2+} by altering the transmembrane flux of Ca^{2+}. However, these data do not indicate the existence of effects of vasopressin on plasma membrane Ca^{2+} permeability or Ca^{2+} pump activity. Recently, there have been reports of a small inhibition of $(Ca^{2+}-Mg^{2+})$ATPase in plasma membranes isolated from hepatocytes treated with vasopressin (20,21). More striking is the inhibition of Ca^{2+} transport in plasma membranes from vasopressin-treated livers observed by Prpić et al. (21). This inhibition is maximal (50%) after 3 min of hormone exposure and is detectable at 1 min. Its concentration-dependence on vasopressin (10^{-10} - 10^{-9} M) is similar to that for other biological parameters e.g. cytosolic Ca^{2+} and phosphorylase a.

Inhibition of the plasma membrane Ca^{2+} pump would be expected to result in an elevation of cytosolic Ca^{2+} which would be maintained since it would not depend on limited intracellular Ca^{2+} stores. In view of its apparently slow onset relative to intracellular Ca^{2+} mobilization, inhibition of the Ca^{2+} pump is probably not involved in the initial hormone responses which occur within seconds and which are associated with a very large efflux of Ca^{2+}.

V. ROLE OF CYTOSOLIC Ca^{2+} IN THE PHYSIOLOGICAL RESPONSES TO CALCIUM-DEPENDENT HORMONES

It is generally accepted that the activation of liver phosphorylase by Ca^{2+}-dependent hormones is due to the rise in cytosolic Ca^{2+} which stimulates phosphorylase b kinase. This kinase has been purified to homogeneity from rat liver in a high (1.3 million) M_r form with an $\alpha 4 \beta 4 \gamma 4 \delta 4$ subunit structure and contains the Ca^{2+}-dependent regulatory protein calmodulin as the δ subunit (22). It is stimulated by an increase in Ca^{2+} concentration from 0.1 μM to 1 μM which is approximately the range through which Ca^{2+}-dependent hormones increase cytosolic Ca^{2+} in liver (3). Further evidence that phosphorylase kinase mediates the effects of Ca^{2+}-dependent hormones on phosphorylase comes from studies with gsd/gsd rats. These animals have a glycogen storage disease due to lack of hepatic phosphorylase b kinase, and hepatocytes prepared from them

show no phosphorylase response to vasopressin or phenylephrine
(23).

   Ca^{2+}-dependent hormones also inactivate glycogen synthase
in liver (24) and there is evidence that phosphorylase _b_
kinase is the Ca^{2+}-sensitive enzyme involved. This enzyme
phosphorylates and inactivates glycogen synthase (25) although
it is considerably more active towards phosphorylase _b_.
Phosphorylase _b_ kinase can also act indirectly by increasing
phosphorylase _a_ which is an inhibitor of liver glycogen
synthase phosphatase (26). Inhibition of this phosphatase
would enhance the ability of protein kinases to phosphorylate
and inactivate the synthase.

   A Ca^{2+}-calmodulin-dependent protein kinase with activity
towards glycogen synthase has been purified from liver (27,28)
and also identified in muscle and brain (29,30). Its physiological substrates are not fully defined, but it can also act
on myosin light chains from smooth muscle (28) and
microtubule-associated proteins and protein 1 from brain (29).
Although the enzyme has been proposed to play a major role in
Ca^{2+} regulation of liver glycogen synthase (27,31), studies
with calmodulin and calmodulin antagonists in isolated rat
liver cells and liver extracts (26,32) do not support such a
role in this species.

   Another Ca^{2+}-sensitive enzyme which could be involved in
the effects of Ca^{2+}-dependent hormones on liver glycogen
synthase is the Ca^{2+}-phospholipid-dependent protein kinase
discovered by Nishizuka and associates (33,34). However,
although this enzyme phosphorylates liver and muscle glycogen
synthase, it does not cause any inactivation (25).

   In comparison to the situation with the enzymes of glycogen metabolism, the molecular mechanisms involved in the
effects of Ca^{2+}-dependent hormones on other physiological
parameters in liver are less clear. These effects include
changes in gluconeogenesis (35), respiration (36), fatty acid
oxidation (37), amino acid transport (38), K^+ fluxes (39),
branched chain -keto acid oxidation (40) lipogenesis (41) and
the synthesis of certain enzymes of amino acid metabolism
(42). Many of these effects have been shown to require Ca^{2+}
(1) but the role of Ca^{2+} is generally unclear.

   The stimulation of gluconeogenesis by Ca^{2+}-dependent hormones may involve several mechanisms, as is the case for glucagon. Ca^{2+}-dependent hormones have been shown to
phosphorylate and inhibit pyruvate kinase (43) and this probably contributes to the stimulation of gluconeogenesis. The
phosphorylation of pyruvate kinase has been reported to be
Ca^{2+}-dependent (43), but the Ca^{2+}-sensitive protein kinase or
phosphoprotein phosphatase involved is unknown. Other changes
which may be involved in the stimulation of gluconeogenesis by
Ca^{2+}-dependent hormones are an increase in mitochondrial pyru-

vate carboxylation (44) and increased mitochondrial oxidation of cytosolic reduced pyridine nucleotide through Ca^{2+} stimulation of mitochondrial glycerol-3-P dehydrogenase (45).

The stimulation of respiration by the Ca^{2+}-dependent hormones could be due in part to increased oxidation of cytosolic NADH as described above. Other possibilities are Ca^{2+} activation of the 2-oxoglutarate and pyruvate dehydrogenase complexes and of NAD^{+}-linked isocitrate dehydrogenase (46). Pyruvate dehydrogenase activity is increased in hepatocytes by Ca^{2+}-dependent hormones (17,46), but the postulated changes in the other two enzymes are speculative.

The stimulation of fatty acid oxidation to CO_2 induced by Ca^{2+}-dependent hormones in hepatocytes from fed rats (47) may be related to their antiketogenic action (37). The effect is not due to alterations in fatty acid esterification or β-oxidation, but is apparently due to increased citric acid cycle activity (47). The specific mitochondrial enzyme reactions involved are unknown.

The reported effects of Ca^{2+}-dependent hormones on lipogenesis have not been consistent (41,48). α-Adrenergic agonists have been stated to be inhibitory (48) or without effect (41) on hepatic fatty acid synthesis or acetyl-CoA carboxylase, whereas vasopressin has been reported to be stimulatory. A possible resolution of these differences is that the effects of the α-agonists are due mainly to an increase in cAMP (48). In this regard, it has been observed that α_1-adrenergic agonists increase cAMP in the livers of mature rats as opposed to juvenile rats (49), and it has been shown that glucagon and dibutyryl cAMP phosphorylate and inactivate acetyl-CoA carboxylase in hepatocytes (50,51).

Ca^{2+}-dependent hormones have different effects on K^{+} fluxes in liver of different species. In guinea pig, K^{+} efflux is observed and is attributed to a Ca^{2+}-mediated increase in plasma membrane K^{+} permeability (52). In rat, there is a transient influx of K^{+} (9,39) which is postulated to be due to a Ca^{2+}-dependent stimulation of $(Na^{+}$-$K^{+})$ATPase activity (53).

VI. INTRACELLULAR SIGNALLING MECHANISMS OF CALCIUM-DEPENDENT HORMONES

The hepatic receptors for the Ca^{2+}-dependent hormones are located in the plasma membrane as revealed by radioligand binding studies (11,54-56). However, it is not known how activation of these receptors is linked to the cellular Ca^{2+} fluxes induced by the hormones. Since a major factor in the initial rise in cytosolic Ca^{2+} is release of Ca^{2+} from mitochondria, there must be some form of communication between the plasma membrane receptors and these organelles. In addition, there must be some later coupling to the plasma membrane Ca^{2+} pump.

Mitochondria isolated from livers treated with Ca^{2+}-dependent hormones show stable changes in respiration, adenine nucleotides and Ca^{2+} handling (12,57), but the relationship between these changes and those occurring in the intact cells is unclear. With respect to the changes in the plasma membrane Ca^{2+} pump, it is unclear whether these involve the putative cytosolic messenger or a more direct interaction of the receptors with the pump, or are merely secondary to the rise in cytosolic Ca^{2+}.

As will be discussed below, certain products of phosphoinositide metabolism have been proposed as intracellular "second messengers" for the Ca^{2+}-dependent hormones. In addition, Na^+ and H^+ and cyclic GMP have been proposed. However, there is much evidence against a role for Na^+ in liver (58) and no changes in cytosolic or mitochondrial pH have been detected in hepatocytes incubated with phenylephrine (59). Data on the effects of Ca^{2+}-dependent hormones on cyclic GMP levels in liver are inconsistent, and observations in other tissues indicate that the increase in the nucleotide may be the result rather than the cause of the rise in Ca^{2+}.

VII. EFFECTS OF CALCIUM-DEPENDENT HORMONES ON PHOSPHOINOSITIDE METABOLISM

Several studies have shown that Ca^{2+}-dependent hormones stimulate the turnover of phosphatidylinositol and phosphatidylinositol-4,5-bisphosphate in liver (60-63) as in other tissues. It has also been proposed that this turnover plays a primary causal role in the cell Ca^{2+} changes induced by the hormones. Stimulation of the breakdown of phosphatidylinositol in liver by vasopressin and epinephrine has been demonstrated in studies employing isotopic labelling of the phospholipid or chemical measurements. However, the breakdown is relatively slow, i.e. it is not detectable during the first minute (60), whereas Ca^{2+} is mobilized within 2 s (3,4). The breakdown is also Ca^{2+}-dependent and requires higher hormone concentrations than does Ca^{2+} mobilization or phosphorylase activation (4,60). Thus it is unlikely that changes in this particular phospholipid play a primary role in the initial changes in Ca^{2+}.

More recently, attention has been focussed on a more highly phosphorylated derivative of phosphatidylinositol, namely phosphatidylinositol-4,5-bisphosphate, since this compound breaks down more rapidly in hepatocytes in response to Ca^{2+}-dependent hormones than does phosphatidylinositol (61, 62). It has been proposed that the breakdown of this poly-phosphoinositide increases the permeability of the plasma membrane to Ca^{2+} in some undefined manner ("opens Ca^{2+} gates") and/or generates a second messenger which releases intracellular Ca^{2+} (63,64). Two suggested second messengers are inositol 1,4,5-trisphosphate and diacylglycerol, which are the immediate products of phosphatidylinositol-4,5-bisphosphate breakdown by phosphodiesterase. Other possibilities are phosphatidate, derived from diacylglycerol by the action of diacylglycerol kinase, and arachidonate (and its further metabolites) derived from diacylglycerol through lipase action.

As illustrated in Fig. 4, administration of vasopressin to hepatocytes rapidly decreases phosphatidylinositol-4,5-bisphosphate. There is a simultaneous increase in inositol-1,4,5-trisphosphate (4). The effects are detectable within 5 s and persist for 5-10 min (4). This time course of phosphatidylinositol-4,5-bisphosphate breakdown supports the view that it may play a role in Ca^{2+} mobilization. However, studies of concentration-dependence of the effect have given discordant results. In two reports, the breakdown was unaffected by vasopressin concentrations (10^{-10} M – 10^{-9} M) which increase cytosolic Ca^{2+} and activate phosphorylase (4,61). In another report, the dose responses for the breakdown of the phospholipid and for the activation of phosphorylase were well correlated (63). Thus it is not possible at present to define a role for phosphatidylinositol-4,5-bisphosphate turnover in the initial actions of Ca^{2+}-dependent hormones in liver unless it is proposed that only a very small breakdown of the phospholipid is required to cause Ca^{2+} mobilization. Irrespective of the possible role of phosphatidylinositol-4,5-bisphosphate breakdown, there is increasing evidence that inositol-1,4,5-trisphosphate released from the phospholipid acts as a "second messenger". This is because its addition to permeabilized cells and isolated mitochondria and microsomes causes Ca^{2+} release (65-67). In other cells e.g. platelets, it has been proposed that phosphoinositide breakdown generates diacylglycerol which activates a specific protein kinase or is converted to phosphatidate which acts as a Ca^{2+} ionophore. Diacylglycerol has been shown to activate a Ca^{2+}-phospholipid-dependent protein kinase (34) by reducing its requirement for Ca^{2+} to near the cytosolic range (68). This enzyme is present in liver (69) and could therefore play a role in some of the hepatic actions of the Ca^{2+}-dependent hormones. The effect of diacylglycerol to activate the kinase can be mimicked by phorbol esters (70). Addition of these esters to hepatocytes does not reproduce the changes in glycogen metabolism induced by

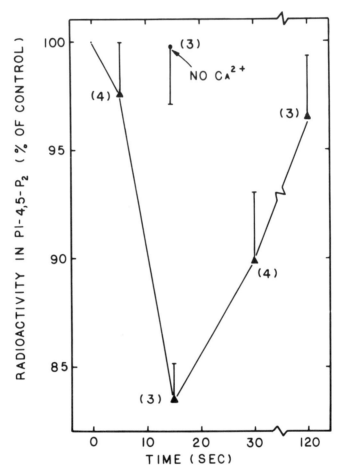

FIGURE 4. Time course of vasopressin-stimulated phospha-
tidylinositol-4,5-bisphosphate (PI-4,5-P$_2$) in hepatocytes
prelabeled with [^{3}H]myo-inositol and exposed to 10^{-8} M
vasopressin. From Rhodes et al. (61)

the Ca^{2+}-dependent hormones (unpublished findings; 71).
However, there is increased phosphorylation of certain cytosolic proteins (71) indicating the presence of endogenous
substrates for the Ca^{2+}-phospholipid-dependent protein kinase.
With respect to phosphatidate or arachidonate playing a
messenger role in liver, Barritt and associates have provided
several lines of evidence against these possibilities (72,73).
    In summary, it appears unlikely that the breakdown of
phosphatidylinositol induced in liver by Ca^{2+}-dependent hormones is responsible for the initial changes in cellular Ca^{2+}
which trigger the biological responses. However, the more

rapidly   occurring   breakdown   of   phosphatidylinositol-4,5-bisphosphate probably plays some role.

VIII. SUMMARY

Calcium-dependent hormones such as norepinephrine and epinephrine (acting via α_1-adrenergic receptors) and vasopressin elicit their biological responses in liver by increasing cytosolic Ca^{2+}. Phosphorylase b kinase is the Ca^{2+}-stimulated, calmodulin-containing enzyme responsible for the activation of glycogen phosphorylase induced by these hormones, and is probably involved in the inactivation of glycogen synthase. However, the Ca^{2+}-sensitive proteins involved in the other physiological changes are presently unknown.

The hormones increase cytosolic Ca^{2+} initially by causing release of the cation from mitochondria and perhaps other intracellular stores. They also inhibit the plasma membrane $(Ca^{2+}-Mg^{2+})$ATPase pump, but this appears to be a more slowly developing effect which functions to prolong the biological responses.

The   hormones   rapidly   stimulate   the   breakdown   of phosphatidylinositol-4,5-bisphosphate and there is increasing evidence that this is causally related to the alterations in Ca^{2+} and other responses.

REFERENCES

1.   Exton, J. H., Mol. Cell. Endocrinol. 23:233 (1981).
2.   Murphy, E., Coll, K., Rich, T. L., and Williamson, J. R., J. Biol. Chem. 255:6600 (1980).
3.   Charest, R., Blackmore, P. F., Berthon, B., and Exton, J. H., J. Biol. Chem. 258:8769 (1983).
4.   Charest, R., Prpič, V., Exton, J. H., and Blackmore, P. F., J. Biol. Chem. 259:(in press) (1984).
5.   Tsien, R. Y., Biochemistry 19:2396 (1980).
6.   Tsien, R. Y., Pozzan, T., and Kirk, T. J., J. Cell Biol. 94:325 (1982).
7.   Assimacopoulos-Jeannet, F. D., Blackmore, P. F., and Exton, J. H., J. Biol. Chem. 252:2662 (1977).
8.   Blackmore, P. F., Brumley, F. T., Marks, J. L., and Exton, J. H., J. Biol. Chem. 253:4851 (1978).
9.   Blackmore, P. F., Dehaye, J. -P., and Exton, J. H., J. Biol. Chem. 254:6945 (1979).
10. Blackmore, P. F., Hughes, B. P., Shuman, E. A., and Exton, J. H., J. Biol. Chem. 257:190 (1982).

11. Dehaye, J. -P., Blackmore, P. F., Venter, J. C., and
    Exton, J. H., J. Biol. Chem. 255:3905 (1980).
12. Dehaye, J. -P., Hughes, B. P., Blackmore, P. F., and
    Exton, J. H., Biochem. J. 194:949 (1981).
13. Barritt, G. J., Parker, J. C., and Wadsworth, J. C.,
    J. Physiol. (Lond.) 312:29 (1981).
14. Babcock, D. F., Chen, J. -L. J., Yip, B. P., and Lardy,
    H. A., J. Biol. Chem. 254:8117 (1979).
15. Studer, R. K., and Borle, A. B., Biochim. Biophys. Acta
    762:302 (1983).
16. Poggioli, J., Berthon, B., and Claret, M., FEBS Lett.
    115:243 (1980).
17. Blackmore, P. F., Hughes, B. P., and Exton, J. H., in
    "Isolation, Characterization and Use of Hepatocytes" (R.
    A. Harris, and N. W. Cornell, eds.), p.433. Elsevier/
    North-Holland Biomedical Press, Amsterdam, 1983.
18. Burgess, G. M., Giraud, F., Poggioli, J., and Claret, M.,
    Biochim. Biophys. Acta 731:387 (1983).
19. Morgan, N. G., Shuman, E. A., Exton, J. H., and
    Blackmore, P. F., J. Biol. Chem. 257:13907 (1982).
20. Lin, S. -H., Wallace, M. A., and Fain, J. N., Fed. Proc.
    41:1458 (1982).
21. Prpic, V., Green, K., Blackmore, P. F., and Exton, J. H.,
    J. Biol. Chem. 259:1382 (1984).
22. Chrisman, T. D., Jordan, J. E., and Exton, J. H., J.
    Biol. Chem. 257:10798 (1982).
23. Blackmore, P. F., and Exton, J. H., Biochem. J. 198:379
    (1981).
24. Strickland, W. G., Blackmore, P. F., and Exton, J. H.,
    Diabetes 29:617 (1980).
25. Imazu, M., Strickland, W. G., Chrisman, T. D., and Exton,
    J. H., J. Biol. Chem. 259:1813 (1984).
26. Strickland, W. G., Imazu, M., Chrisman, T. D., and Exton,
    J. H., J. Biol. Chem. 258:5490 (1983).
27. Payne, M. E., and Soderling, T. R., J. Biol. Chem. 255:
    8054 (1980).
28. Ahmad, Z., DePaoli-Roach, A. P., and Roach, P. J., J.
    Biol. Chem. 257:8348 (1982).
29. Woodgett, J. R., Tonks, N. K., and Cohen, P., FEBS Lett.
    148:5 (1982).
30. Kennedy, M. B., McGuinness, T., and Greengard, P., J.
    Neurosci. 3:818 (1983).
31. Payne, M. E., Schworer, C. M., and Soderling, T. R.,
    J. Biol. Chem. 258:2376 (1983).
32. Blackmore, P. F., El-Refai, M. F., Dehaye, J. -P.,
    Strickland, W. G., Hughes, P. F., and Exton, J. H., FEBS
    Lett. 123:245 (1981).
33. Inoue, M., Kishimoto, A., Takai, Y., and Nishizuka, Y.,
    J. Biol. Chem. 252:7610 (1977).

33. Inoue, M., Kishimoto, A., Takai, Y., and Nishizuka, Y., J. Biol. Chem. 252:7610 (1977).

34. Takai, Y., Kishimoto, A., Iwasa, Y., Kawahara, Y., Mori, T., and Nishizuka, Y., J. Biol. Chem. 254:3692 (1979).

35. Tolbert, M. E. M., Butcher, F. R., and Fain, J. N., J. Biol. Chem. 248:5686 (1973).

36. Sugano, T., Shiota, M., Khono, H., Shimada, M., and Oshino, N., J. Biochem. (Tokyo) 87:465 (1980).

37. Sugden, M. C., Ball, A. J., Ilic, V., and Williamson, D. H., FEBS Lett. 116:37 (1980).

38. LeCam, L., and Freychet, P., Endocrinology 102:379 (1978).

39. Jakob, A., and Diem, S., Biochim. Biophys. Acta 404:57 (1975).

40. Buxton, D., Barron, L. L., and Olson, M. S., J. Biol. Chem. 257:14318 (1982).

41. Assimacopoulos-Jeannet, F., Denton, R. M., and Jeanrenaud, B., Biochem. J. 198:485 (1981).

42. Noda, C., Nakamura, T., and Ichihara, A., J. Biol. Chem. 258:1520 (1983).

43. Garrison, J. C., Borland, M. K., Florio, V. A., and Twible, D. A., J. Biol. Chem. 254:7147 (1979).

44. Garrison, J. C., and Borland, M. K., J. Biol. Chem. 254:1129 (1979).

45. Wernette, M. E., Ochs, R. S., and Lardy, H. A., J. Biol. Chem. 256:12767 (1981).

46. Denton, R. M., McCormack, J. G., and Oviasu, O. A., in "Short-Term Regulation of Liver Metabolism" (L. Hue, and G. Van de Werve, eds.), p.159. Elsevier/North-Holland, Biomedical Press, Amsterdam, 1981.

47. Sugden, M. C., and Watts, D. I., Biochem. J. 212:85 (1983).

48. Ly, S., and Kim, K. -H., J. Biol. Chem. 256:11585 (1981).

49. Morgan, N. G., Blackmore, P. F., and Exton, J. H., J. Biol. Chem. 258:5103 (1983).

50. Witters, L. A., Kowaloff, E. M., and Avruch, J., J. Biol. Chem. 254:245 (1979).

51. Ly, S., and Kim, K. -H., Arch. Biochem. Biophys. 217:251 (1982).

52. Haylett, D. G., and Jenkinson, D. H., J. Physiol. (Lond.) 255:751 (1972).

53. Capiod, T., Berthon, B., Poggioli, J., Burgess, G. M., and Claret, M., FEBS Lett. 141:49 (1982).

54. El-Refai, M. F., Blackmore, P. F., and Exton, J. H., J. Biol. Chem. 254:4375 (1979).

55. Campanile, C. P., Crane, J. K., Peach, M. J., and Garrison, J. C., J. Biol. Chem. 257:4951 (1982).

56. Cantau, B., Keppens, S., DeWulf, H., Jard, S., J. Receptor Res. 1:137 (1980).

57. Taylor, W. M., Prpić, V., Exton, J. H., and Bygrave, F. L., Biochem. J. 188:443 (1980).
58. Hughes, B. P., Blackmore, P. F., and Exton, J. H., FEBS Lett. 121:260 (1980).
59. Strzelecki, T., LaNoue, K. F., and Thomas, J. A., in "Isolation, Characterization and Use of Hepatocytes" (R. A. Harris, and N. W. Cornell, eds.), p.303. Elsevier/North-Holland Biomedical Press, Amsterdam, 1983.
60. Prpić, V., Blackmore, P. F., and Exton, J. H., J. Biol. Chem. 257:11323 (1982).
61. Rhodes, D., Prpić, V., Exton, J. H., and Blackmore, P. F., J. Biol. Chem. 258:2770 (1983).
62. Creba, J. A., Downes, C. P., Hawkins, P. T., Brewster, G., Michell, R. H., and Kirk, C. J., Biochem. J. 212:733 (1983).
63. Thomas, A. P., Marks, J. S., Coll, K. E., and Williamson, J. R., J. Biol. Chem. 258:5716 (1983).
64. Downes, P., and Michell, R. H., Cell Calcium 3:467 (1982).
65. Streb, H., Irvine, R. F., Berridge, M. J., and Schulz, I., Nature 306:67 (1983).
66. Joseph, S. K., Thomas, A. P., Williams, R. J., Irvine, R. F., and Williamson, J. R., J. Biol. Chem. 259:3077 (1984).
67. Thiyagarajah, P., Charest, R., Exton, J. H., and Blackmore, P. F., J. Biol. Chem. (submitted) (1984).
68. Kishimoto, A., Takai, Y., Mori, T., Kikkawa, U., and Nishizuka, Y., J. Biol. Chem. 255:2273 (1980).
69. Kuo, J. F., Anderson, R. G. G., Wise, B. C., Mackerlova, L., Salomonsson, I., Brackett, N. L., Katoh, N., Shoji, M., and Wrenn, R. W., Proc. Natl. Acad. Sci. U.S.A. 77:7039 (1980).
70. Castagna, M., Takai, Y., Kaibuchi, K., Sano, K., Kikkawa, U., and Nishizuka, Y., J. Biol. Chem. 257:7847 (1982).
71. Garrison, J. C., in "Isolation, Characterization and Use of Hepatocytes" (R. A. Harris, and N. W. Cornell, eds.), p.551, Elsevier/North-Holland Biomedical Press, Amsterdam, 1983.
72. Barritt, G. J., Dalton, K. A., and Whiting, J. A., FEBS Lett. 125:137 (1981).
73. Whiting, J. A., and Barritt, G. J., Biochem. J. 206:121 (1982).

ISLET-ACTIVATING PROTEIN, PERTUSSIS TOXIN, AS A PROBE FOR RECEPTOR-MEDIATED SIGNAL TRANSDUCTION[1]

Michio Ui
Toshiaki Katada
Toshihiko Murayama
Tsutomu Nakamura

Department of Physiological Chemistry
Faculty of Pharmaceutical Sciences
Hokkaido University
Sapporo

I. ISLET-ACTIVATING PROTEIN AS AN EXOTOXIN PRODUCED BY BORDETELLA PERTUSSIS

A rat injected once intraperitoneally with pertussis vaccine (10^{11} organisms per 100 g of body wt) displayed, despite normoglycemia and normoinsulinemia in the fasted or non-stimulated state, much greater insulinemic response to feeding or an injection of insulin secretagogues than did an unvaccinated control rat (1). In addition, epinephrine-induced hyperglycemia usually observed within 2 hr was no longer seen in rats that had received a single injection of pertussis vaccine 2 to 7 days before (1,2). This blockade of epinephrine hyperglycemia was invariably associated with striking hyperinsulinemia, indicating that the catecholamine was capable of stimulating insulin secretion in the vaccine-treated rats (2).

The manner in which pertussis vaccine durably enhances the insulin secretory response of rats was further studied in perfusion experiments using pancreatic organs isolated from

[1]This work was supported by research grants from the Scientific Research Fund of the Ministry of Education, Science and Culture, Japan.

vaccine-treated or control rats (3). Results clearly showed that α-adrenergic inhibition of insulin secretion was completely reversed and β-adrenergic stimulation of the secretion was greatly potentiated by prior vaccine treatment of the pancreas-donor rats. Glucose-, glucagon- or arginine-induced insulin secretion in vitro was also enhanced by the pertussis vaccine treatment in vivo (3). These early studies in our laboratory were thus strongly suggestive of the presence of a new factor in the vaccine that modifies receptor-mediated responses of pancreatic islets, and encouraged our pursuit of further experiments aimed at isolation of this factor. The factor was soon purified as a homogeneous protein with a molecular weight (M_r) of 117,000 (4), and was termed an islet-activating protein (IAP).

All of the above-mentioned effects of pertussis vaccine on rats were reproduced by minute doses of IAP. Rat insulin secretory response to glucose load was enhanced 10- to 12-fold during 2 to 7 days after a single intravenous injection of 1 μg of IAP (4). In addition, it produced marked lymphocytosis in rats, mice and rabbits, increased the number of mice that were killed by a semi-lethal dose of histamine and induced hemagglutination in vitro (5). Thus, IAP must be identical with the pertussis toxin that has been extensively studied by a number of investigators as a lymphocytosis-promoting factor, a histamine-sensitizing factor or a hemagglutinin (6,7). Our own studies have therefore added an important biological activity, an islet-activating activity, to this toxin, together with proposal of a productive purification procedure for this important material from the culture medium of whooping cough bacteria.

The action of IAP was characterized by its slow onset as well as by its long duration. Such was the case with its action on a variety of cell types in vitro as shown below, suggesting that the exposure of cells to IAP results in an irreversible modification of the cellular component(s) that should play a pivotal role in development of cellular functions.

II. ISLET-ACTIVATING PROTEIN AS A SPECIFIC MODIFIER OF THE RECEPTOR-ADENYLATE CYCLASE SYSTEM

Stimulation of insulin secretion by a β-adrenergic agonist, glucagon or glucose was associated with an increase in the content of cyclic AMP in islet cells. Likewise, inhibition of insulin secretion by an α-adrenergic agonist resulted from a decrease in islet cell cyclic AMP. Thus, cyclic AMP appears to act as a second messenger in the receptor-mediated

regulation of insulin secretion. Modification by IAP of insulin secretory responses was invariably associated with changes
in the cellular content of cyclic AMP in the same direction
(8-10). These changes were observed in the presence of an
inhibitor of cyclic nucleotide phosphodiesterase, suggesting
that IAP modifies receptor-mediated regulation of adenylate
cyclase activity. Actually, the magnitude of α-adrenergic
inhibition of adenylate cyclase activity was much less in
membranes from IAP-treated islets than in membranes from non-
treated islets (11).

Not only islet cells but also cells of other types were
susceptible to IAP action. Exposure of rat heart cells to IAP
for 3 hr resulted in marked potentiation of β-adrenergic
receptor-mediated increases in cyclic AMP and total aboli-
tion of muscarinic cholinergic receptor- or adenosine (A_1)
receptor-mediated decreases in the nucleotide (12). The
decrease in the cyclic nucleotide via adenosine P-sites was
not affected by the IAP treatment (13), indicating that
coupling of membrane receptors with adenylate cyclase is the
site of IAP action. Stimulation by GTP of membrane adenylate
cyclase activity was also enhanced by prior exposure to
IAP of the cells from which the membrane was prepared (14), in
accord with the currently accepted view that guanine
nucleotide regulatory protein (N) is involved in the membrane
receptor-adenylate cyclase coupling. The cells that have
thus far been found to be susceptible to IAP are: rat
islet cells ($α_2$-adrenergic receptors) (11), rat heart cells
(β-adrenergic, muscarinic and adenosine (A_1) receptors)
(12), rat glioma C6 cells (-adrenergic receptors) (14),
rat glioma x mouse neuroblastoma NG108-15 hybrid cells
(prostaglandin E, $α_2$-adrenergic, muscarinic and opiate
receptors) (15), rat adipocytes (glucagon, β-adrenergic,
adenosine (A_1) and nicotinic acid receptors) (16), hamster
adipocytes (β- and $α_2$-adrenergic receptors) (17), mouse 3T3
fibroblasts (18) and rat mast cells (19). The receptor-
mediated inhibition of adenylate cyclase was reversed, or
activation was enhanced, after IAP treatment of the cells.

III. ISLET-ACTIVATING PROTEIN AS A CATALYST
OF ADP-RIBOSYLATION OF A MEMBRANE PROTEIN

Although the membrane receptor-adenylate cyclase system
appeared to be the target site of IAP action, no significant
change had been observed in the adenylate cyclase activity
upon direct exposure of isolated membranes to IAP. Long-term
exposure of intact cells to IAP in vitro or injection of the
toxin into the animal in vivo one or more days before was

indispensable to the observation of IAP action. It was later found, however, that brief exposure of C6 cell membranes to IAP resulted in rapid enhancement of GTP-dependent adenylate cyclase activity only if the incubation medium was fortified with NAD (20). Under these conditions radioactivity was incorporated from ^{32}P-labeled NAD into the membrane protein with an M_r value of 41,000 (Fig. 1). The adenine (Lane 2 in Fig. 1) and the pyrophosphate (Lane 3) moieties of NAD were incorporated into the protein, but no radioactivity was detected when the nicotinamide moiety of NAD was labeled with ^{14}C (Lane 1). Moreover, ^{32}P once incorporated into the M_r=41,000 protein was lost, as 5'-AMP, upon incubation of the labeled membranes with snake venom phosphodiesterase (Lane 5 in Fig. 1). Thus, IAP catalyzed the transfer of the ADP-ribose moiety of NAD into the membrane M_r=41,000 protein.

The degree of IAP-catalyzed ADP-ribosylation of the M_r=41,000 protein in membranes was well correlated with the increment in GTP-dependent adenylate cyclase in the same membranes (21). Such was the case with the membranes isolated from IAP-treated cells: during long-term exposure of intact cells to IAP, the ADP-ribose moiety of the intracellular non-radioactive NAD was transferred to the M_r=41,000 protein, as revealed by the failure of IAP, again added to the medium for the subsequent incubation of membranes isolated from the thus IAP-treated cells, to label the same protein by radioactive NAD (21). Tryptic digestion of the ADP-ribosylated membranes resulted in decomposition of the M_r=41,000 protein to peptides with smaller M_r values. The digestion pattern was profoundly affected by the prior incubation of membranes with Gpp(NH)p, a hydrolysis-resistant analogue of GTP, or NaF. Since both Gpp(NH)p and fluoride were specific ligands of the guanine nucleotide regulatory proteins (N), it is reasonable to assume that the M_r=41,000 protein is one of its subunits (21).

Further studies with 3T3 cells (18), rat adipocytes (16) and NG108-15 hybrid cells (15) revealed that the site of action of IAP is N_i, the regulatory protein that is involved in receptor-mediated inhibition of adenylate cyclase. IAP-catalyzed ADP-ribosylation of the M_r=41,000 protein gives rise to a complete loss of the N_i function to communicate between inhibitory receptors and the catalytic unit (C) of the cyclase (15-18). The IAP substrate is the α-subunit of N_i, whereas the substrate protein (M_r=45,000) for cholera toxin-catalyzed ADP-ribosylation is the α-subunit of N_s that is involved in receptor-linked activation of adenylate cyclase (22).

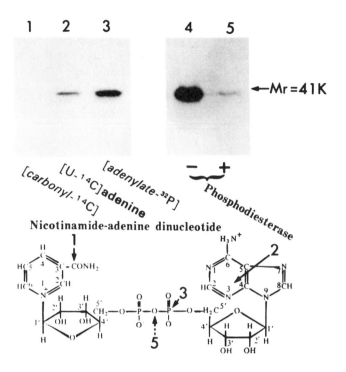

FIGURE 1.   ADP-ribosylation of the membrane M_r=41,000 protein by IAP.   Membranes from rat C6 glioma cells were incubated for 10 min with IAP (25 µg/ml) and 125 µM (50 mCi/mmol)
radioactive NAD as indicated for lanes 1-3 and with 10 µM
[α-^{32}P]NAD (5 Ci/mmol) for lanes 4 and 5.   The labeled membranes were then dissolved in NaDodSO₄ and submitted to
NaDodSO₄-polyacrylamide gel electrophoresis.   Autoradiographic
pattern obtained by exposure of the gel to X-film for 24 hr is
shown.   For lanes 1-3, the position of label in the structure
of NAD is shown by arrows below.   For lane 5, the labeled
membranes were incubated for 2 hr with snake venom phosphodiesterase which hydrolyzes the phosphate bond as shown by an
arrow-5.

IV. ISLET-ACTIVATING PROTEIN AS ONE OF THE A-B TOXINS

IAP is a hexamer with the M_r value of 117,000 and consists
of five dissimilar subunits which are termed S_1 to S_5 in the
order of their molecular weights (23).   Its subunit assembly
is such that the biggest subunit, S_1, is noncovalently associated with the residual   pentamer which is an association

product of two dimers, dimer-1 (S_2 plus S_4) and dimer-2 (S_3 plus S_4), via the smallest subunit, S_5. The native IAP is readily dissociated into S_1 and the pentamer during short-term exposure to 5 M urea. S_1 is an enzyme catalyzing the transfer of the ADP-ribose moiety of the membrane M_r=41,000 protein or hydrolysis of NAD to ADP-ribose and nicotinamide in the absence of cellular components after reductive cleavage of its intrapeptide disulfide bonds by dithiothreitol (24). The native IAP did not display such NAD-glycohydrolase activity. Thus, S_1 is the A (Active) protomer. The A protomer was without effect as such on intact cells of any type which were susceptible to the native IAP, an association product of the A protomer and the pentamer. The pentamer was a competitive inhibitor of the native IAP acting on intact cells, clearly indicating that the native IAP is attached to the cell surface via its pentamer moiety (25). Thus, the pentamer should be a B (Binding) oligomer, and IAP is one of the A-B toxins according to the definition by Gill (26).

It is now established that the IAP molecule enters the cell after its binding, via its B oligomer moiety, to a particular receptor site on the cell surface. During, or immediately after, penetration across the plasma membrane, IAP undergoes "processing" to liberate its A protomer moiety which is readily converted to its active reduced form before catalyzing ADP-ribosylation of the membrane M_r=41,000 protein, an α-subunit of N_i. The definite lag time that invariably precedes the onset of the IAP action on intact cells (27) reflects the time required for such transportation and processing of the IAP molecule in the vicinity of the plasma membrane.

V. ISLET-ACTIVATING PROTEIN STABILIZES N_i IN ITS INACTIVE STATE, WHILE CHOLERA TOXIN STABILIZES N_s IN ITS ACTIVE STATE

Cholera toxin-catalyzed ADP-ribosylation of the α-subunit of N_s is known to result in the inhibition of GTP hydrolysis that should otherwise occur at the GTP binding sites thereon. IAP-catalyzed ADP-ribosylation of the α-subunit of N_i would possibly exert a similar influence on the function of the α-subunit, since opiate receptor-mediated GTPase activity was also inhibited by the A protomer of IAP (28) or IAP itself (29) in membranes of NG108-15 cells. This possibility, however, has been denied by our recent experiments in which the GTP-GDP exchange reaction, rather than GTPase activity, on N was estimated under the influence of coupled receptor stimulation (17).

Incubation of membranes with [^{3}H]GTP resulted in its binding to the specific GTP sites on N in exchange for endogenously bound GDP, only if receptors coupled to the N were simultaneously stimulated by the addition of a receptor agonist. Excess [^{3}H]GTP was then washed away by further incubation of the labeled membranes in the fresh medium containing non-radioactive GTP and a receptor antagonist. During this washing procedure, [^{3}H]GTP bound to N was hydrolyzed to [^{3}H]GDP. The subsequent incubation of thus prepared [^{3}H]GDP-labeled membranes with non-radioactive GTP (or Gpp(NH)p) in the presence of a receptor agonist provoked rapid release of [^{3}H]GDP which serves as a good measure of receptor-mediated activation of coupled N.

In the case of membranes from rat or hamster adipocytes, [^{3}H]GDP bound as a result of stimulation of β-adrenergic receptors was released during the subsequent incubation in response not only to a β-agonist itself but also to glucagon or secretin, agonists of other "activatory" receptors involved in adenylate cyclase activation via N_s. It was not released, however, if $α_2$-adrenergic, prostaglandin E or adenosine receptors ("inhibitory" receptors), which are involved in the cyclase inhibition via N_i, were instead stimulated (17). ADP-ribosylation of N_s by cholera toxin resulted, but ADP-ribosylation of N_i by IAP did not, in [^{3}H]GDP release from these membranes without stimulation of any activatory receptor. Receptor-mediated [^{3}H]GDP release from these membranes was unaffected by IAP. On the other hand, stimulation of $α_2$-adrenergic receptors labeled hamster adipocyte membranes with [^{3}H]GTP. [^{3}H]GDP release from these membranes was promoted not only by an α-agonist itself but also by agonists of other inhibitory receptors. It was not promoted by any of the agonists of activatory receptors. If these [^{3}H]GTP-labeled membranes were ADP-ribosylated by IAP during the washing procedure, however, further addition of agonists of inhibitory receptors failed to promote [^{3}H]GDP release. Cholera toxin, unlike IAP, was without effect in this regard. Thus, these data indicate that all the activatory receptors are linked to a common pool of the α-subunit of N_s, the specific target site of cholera toxin, while all the inhibitory receptors are coupled to a common pool of the α-subunit of N_i, which is a distinctly different entity from the α-subunit of N_s and is selectively susceptible to the A protomer of IAP.

ADP-ribosylation of N_s by cholera toxin stabilizes its α-subunit in an active state in the sense that the GTP sites thereon are "spontaneously" occupied by GTP without stimulation of coupled activatory receptors. In sharp contrast, ADP-ribosylation of N_i by IAP freezes its α-subunit in such an inactive state that stimulation of coupled inhibitory receptors fails to convert it to the GTP-bound active form. The inhibition of opiate receptor-linked GTPase by IAP (28,29) must result from such blockade of communication between receptors and N_i, while cholera toxin-induced inhibition of GTPase may reflect the maintenance of the active state of N_s.

VI. ISLET-ACTIVATING PROTEIN AS A PROMISING PROBE FOR POSSIBLE INVOLVEMENT OF THE NUCLEOTIDE REGULATORY PROTEIN IN RECEPTOR MEDIATED PHOSPHOLIPID TURNOVER AND CALCIUM FLUX

Stimulation of certain membrane receptors gives rise to activation of phospholipase(s), rather than adenylate cyclase, leading to membrane phospholipid turnover and transmembrane Ca^{2+} flux. Some of these receptors, e.g., muscarinic cholinergic ones, are also linked to adenylate cyclase in an inhibitory fashion, suggesting that these two different systems of signal transduction might be mutually interrelated. IAP, a specific modifier of N_i involved in receptor-mediated inhibition of adenylate cyclase, would serve as a tool in the search for the role of the nucleotide regulatory protein in receptor-mediated phospholipase activation and Ca^{2+} translocation.

Membrane receptors, such as those for compound 48/80, IgE or somatostatin, are responsible for histamine release from mast cells. Histamine release arising from stimulation of these receptors was efficiently prevented by the prior treatment of the cells with small amounts of IAP (19). In contrast, IAP was without effect on A23187-induced histamine release. The dose- and time-dependence of the inhibition of compound 48/80-induced histamine release is illustrated in Fig. 2. IAP became effective after a lag period, which was apparently shortened by increasing the toxin concentration from 0.1 to 10 ng/ml. This is characteristic of the A-B toxin and indicates that the inhibition of histamine release reflects the action of the A protomer of IAP occurring after its penetration across the plasma membrane. In fact, ADP-ribosylation was observed in a protein band with an $M_r=41,000$ (data not shown), but the inhibition was not associated with an increase in the cellular content of cyclic AMP (19). Compound 48/80-induced histamine release was preceded by the incorporation of ^{32}P into the phosphatidic acid, phosphatidylinositol and phosphatidylcholine fractions. In cells treated with IAP, ^{32}Pi was incorporated into both phosphatidic acid and phosphatidylinositol fractions at essentially the same rate as in the control cells not treated with the toxin. The ^{32}P-labeling of phosphatidylcholine, however, was suppressed by IAP (30). Probably, this action of IAP reflects the inhibition of phospholipase A_2 that hydrolyzes

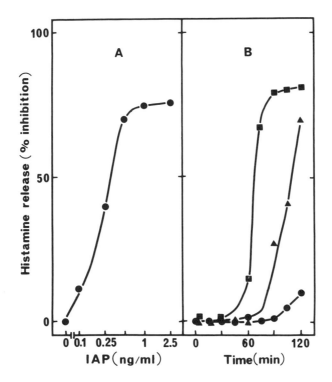

FIGURE 2. Inhibition by IAP of histamine release from mast cells in vitro in response to compound 48/80. Mast cells were exposed to various concentrations of IAP for 2 hr (A), or to 0.1 (●), 1 (▲) or 10 (■) ng/ml of IAP for various lengths of time (B). These cells were then incubated with 0.5 μg/ml of compound 48/80 for 10 min to measure histamine release. The percent inhibition caused by IAP was calculated, and the mean value from duplicate observations is shown in each panel.

phosphatidylcholine preferentially, since IAP was effective in inhibiting the release of arachidonate and its metabolites from the cells that had been labeled with [14C]arachidonic acids (30). The largest radioactivity was found in the phosphatidylcholine fraction. Arachidonic acid release as induced by A23187 was not affected by IAP under the same conditions.

In the case of 3T3 fibroblasts in which the membrane M_r=41,000 protein, the α-subunit of N_i, is ADP-ribosylated by IAP (18), the addition of thrombin resulted in a sharp decrease in cellular cyclic AMP content. The inhibition was completely reversed by prior treatment of the cells with IAP, providing convincing evidence for the view that stimulation of thrombin receptors inhibits adenylate cyclase via N_i (Table I). Interestingly, the thrombin-induced inhibition of adenylate cyclase was associated with phosphatidylinositol (and polyphosphophosphatidylinositol) hydrolysis as revealed by the discharge of preloaded [^{3}H]inositol. Arachidonic acid was also released in response to thrombin (Table I). It is likely, therefore, that thrombin receptors in 3T3 cells are linked to phospholipase C and A_2 activation as well as adenylate cyclase inhibition via N_i. It should be noted that the prior treatment of cells with IAP was very effective in abolishing the receptor-mediated arachidonic acid release but did not alter the degree of phosphatidylinositol decomposition. Metabolism of phosphatidylinositol produces phosphatidic acid which acts as a Ca^{2+}-ionophore. Arachidonic acid will then be released as a result of Ca^{2+} activation of phospholipase A_2.

TABLE I.   Decreases in Cyclic AMP, Release of Arachidonate and Breakdown of Phosphatidylinositol in 3T3 Cells Exposed to IAP

Addition	IAP	Decrease in Cyclic AMP	Arachidonate Release	Inositol Release
		(% of control)		
Thrombin	–	71	195	176
(1 μunit/ml)	+	10	109	177
Phosphatidic	–	82	184	n.d.
acid (30 μg/ml)	+	7	103	n.d.
A23187	–	63	262	274
(10 μM)	+	58	338	281

To the culture medium were added [^{14}C]arachidonic acid (0.5 μCi/dish), [^{3}H]inositol (0.5 μCi/dish) and IAP (100 ng/ml). Sixteen hr after the addition of the radioactive precursors and 3 hr after IAP, a monolayer of 3T3 cells was washed with Krebs-Ringer-Hepes solution 3 times and then incubated for 10 min in the fresh medium containing 20 μM arachidonic acid and 0.5 mM inositol with the additions indicated. The values (means of duplicate observations) are the changes induced by the addition: the percent inhibition in cyclic AMP and the percent increase in arachidonic acid and inositol release. n.d.: not determined.

In fact, the addition of phosphatidic acid to 3T3 cells promoted arachidonate release and also decreased the cyclic AMP
content, probably due to Ca^{2+}-induced inhibition of adenylate
cyclase. These effects of phosphatidic acid were no longer
observable in IAP-treated cells (Table I). In sharp contrast,
the similar effects of A23187 were totally insensitive to IAP.
Thrombin stimulates ^{86}Rb uptake into 3T3 cells. This ^{86}Rb
uptake was antagonized by ouabain, but not affected by
the prior treatment of the cells with IAP (data not shown).
Thus, not all the functions of thrombin receptors were
suppressed by IAP. Based on the foregoing data, a possible
involvement of the IAP-susceptible α-subunit of N_i in the
receptor-phospholipid-Ca^{2+} system is suggested in Fig. 3. As
shown, phosphatidic acid-induced Ca^{2+} entry might be supported
by N_i, since this was IAP-sensitive but A23187-induced entry
was not. Alternatively, it is possible to assume that the
-subunit of N_i might act as an activator of phospholipase A_2
in the presence of a moderate concentration of intracellular
Ca^{2+} as induced by phosphatidic acid. In any case, further
use of IAP will provide insight into the mechanism underlying
the receptor-linked signal transduction.

An Involvement of Ni (αi = IAP Substrate) in the Phospholipid–Ca System

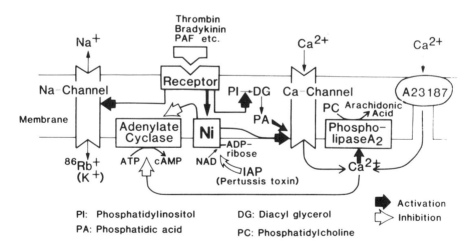

FIGURE 3. A hypothetical scheme for an involvement of
IAP-sensitive N_i in receptor-mediated signal transduction in
3T3 fibroblasts.

REFERENCES

1. Sumi, T., and Ui, M., Endocrinology 97:352 (1975).
2. Katada, T., and Ui, M., Biochim. Biophys. Acta 421:57 (1976).
3. Katada, T., and Ui., M., Endocrinology 101:1247 (1977).
4. Yajima, M., Hosoda, K., Kanbayashi, Y., Nakamura, T., Nogimori, K., Nakase, Y., and Ui, M., J. Biochem. 83:295 (1978).
5. Yajima, M., Hosoda, K., Kanbayashi, Y., Nakamura, T., Takahashi, I., and Ui, M., J. Biochem. 83:305 (1978).
6. Pittman, M., Rev. Infect. Dis. 1:401 (1979).
7. Wardlaw, A. C., and Parton, R., Pharmacol. Ther. 19:1 (1983).
8. Katada, T., and Ui, M., J. Biol. Chem. 254:469 (1979).
9. Katada, T., and Ui, M., Endocrinology 104:1822 (1979).
10. Katada, T., and Ui, M., J. Biochem. 89:979 (1981).
11. Katada, T., and Ui, M., J. Biol. Chem. 256:8310 (1981).
12. Hazeki, O., and Ui, M., J. Biol. Chem. 256:2856 (1981).
13. Hazeki, O., Katada, T., Kurose, H., and Ui, M., in "Physiology and Pharmacology of Adenosine" (J. W. Daly, Y. Kuroda, J. W. Phillis, H. Shimizu, and M. Ui, eds.), p.41. Raven Press, New York, 1983.
14. Katada, T., Amano, T., and Ui, M., J. Biol. Chem. 257:3739 (1982).
15. Kurose, H., Katada, T., Amano, T., and Ui, M., J. Biol. Chem. 258:4870 (1983).
16. Murayama, T., and Ui, M., J. Biol. Chem. 258:3319 (1983).
17. Murayama, T., and Ui, M., J. Biol. Chem. 259:761 (1984).
18. Murayama, T., Katada, T., and Ui, M., Arch. Biochem. Biophys. 221:381 (1983).
19. Nakamura, T., and Ui, M., Biochem. Pharmacol. 32:3435 (1983).
20. Katada, T., and Ui, M., Proc. Natl. Acad. Sci. USA 79:3129 (1982).
21. Katada, T., and Ui, M., J. Biol. Chem. 257:7210 (1982).
22. Bokoch, G. M., Katada, T., Northup, J. K., Hewlett, E. L., and Gilman, A. G., J. Biol. Chem. 258:2072 (1983).
23. Tamura, M., Nogimori, K., Murai, S., Yajima, M., Ito, K., Katada, T., Ui, M., and Ishii, S., Biochemistry 21:5516 (1982).
24. Katada, T., and Ui, M., Arch. Biochem. Biophys. 224:290 (1983).
25. Tamura, M., Nogimori, K., Yajima, M., Ase, K., and Ui, M., J. Biol. Chem. 258:6756 (1983).
26. Gill, M., in "Bacterial Toxins and Cell Membranes" (J. Jeljaszewicz, and T. Wadstrom, eds.), p.291. Academic Press, New York, 1978.

27. Katada, T., and Ui, M., J. Biol. Chem. 255:9580 (1980).
28. Ui, M., Katada, T., Murayama, T., Kurose, H., Yajima, M., Tamura, M., Nakamura, T., and Nogimori, K., in "Advances in Cyclic Nucleotide Research", Vol. 17 (P. Greengard, G. A. Robison, and R. Paoletti, eds.), p. 145. Raven Press, New York, 1984.
29. Burns, D. L., Hewlett, E. L., Moss, J., and Vaughan, M., J. Biol. Chem. 258:1435 (1983).
30. Nakamura, T., and Ui, M., Submitted for publication.

FUNCTIONAL PROPERTIES OF CALCIUM CHANNELS

Arthur M. Brown

Department of Physiology & Biophysics,
University of Texas Medical Branch
Galveston, Texas

I. INTRODUCTION

Membrane calcium channels serve as the link between out-side events usually electrical, sometimes chemical, which impinge upon a cell and the response of the cell to these events. The channels act as triggers because of the rela-tively huge amounts of Ca ion each channel lets into the cell. This is particularly true for small cells or cells in which the surface area to volume ratio is large. Take a small spherical cell, 10 μm in diameter. At 10^{-8} M intracellular Ca activity, the cell contains about 3,000 free Ca ions. A single Ca channel at zero mV membrane potential has a current amplitude of about 0.5 pA (in 40mM Ca_o) and an average life-time of 1.0 msec. One event therefore allows about 3,000 Ca ions to enter. If current flow occurs according to the con-stant field equation the corrected value at physiological Ca_o would be about 150 (1). Given a Ca channel density of about 1 μm^{-2} (2), a probability of opening of 0.1 (2) and a current pulse of 1 msec duration, about 5,000 Ca ions would enter the cell. An estimate of changes in Ca_i between 0.5 and 1.0 log units would likely encompass most possibilities. These changes correspond to direct measurements of Ca_i during Ca current flow made with a variety of techniques in larger cells. Since Ca ions regulate a large number of cell func-tions it is not surprising that cells respond dramatically

---

[1]This work was supported in part by NIH grants HS11453 and HL25145.

CALCIUM REGULATION
IN BIOLOGICAL SYSTEMS

during and following an action potential. Thus the trigger action of Ca ions resides in the gating of the membrane Ca channels by membrane potential or chemicals including, as we shall see, Ca ions itself.

II. BACKGROUND

The functional responses have been studied mainly using electrophysiological methods and a historical account of these studies has been provided (3-5). A progression that is common to all electrophysiological studies may be described. First came studies on the changes in membrane potential which could be inferred as being due to Ca currents (3-5). Next came the study of whole cell or macroscopic Ca currents under voltage clamp (6-8). The voltage clamp experiments proved difficult for three reasons because: (i) cells being examined were not as easy to control as the squid giant axon used in the study of Na and K channels; (ii) the time course of other cell currents notably K currents, some of them even Ca-activated, overlapped the Ca currents and made separation of the Ca current difficult; and (iii) the very low level of intracellular Ca, Ca_i, made measurement of the reversal potential very imprecise particularly given the presence of contaminating outward currents. The reversal potential measurement is very important for estimates of relative membrane permeabilities of different ionic species and selectivity studies on the Ca channel have been hindered because the measurement is so difficult. These problems have persisted although the introduction of methods for dialyzing neurons (7,9,10), favorite cells for the study of Ca currents, have improved the situation considerably, particularly as regards the first two difficulties listed. Voltage clamp studies of internally perfused neurons were followed by measurement of small current fluctuations or noise arising from either the entire somal membrane (11,12) or from large patches several hundred micra in area (11,12). These allowed estimates of single channel conductance which turned out to be too low, and channel density which turned out to be too high. A similar sequence of methodological improvements is not unknown for other membrane channels. However the most notable advances in recent years have followed application of the gigaseal patch clamp method to the study of single Ca channels in a variety of excitable membranes (13-17). The reason is quite simple: many of the uncertainties in recordings from whole cells such as contamination with other currents and adequacy of voltage control are obviated. However the method has limitations largely because of the low signal to noise ratio of unitary Ca currents. The bandwidth is limited to 1.0 to 1.5 kHz, the potential range to about −25 to +5 mV, and most studies use isotonic Ba to enhance unitary currents. These bandwidth limitations are not present in adequately designed voltage clamp experiments (18, 19). Therefore it is important to use a variety of methods each selected for the particular experimental requirements.

The gigaseal method may also be used in the single electrode voltage clamp mode by bursting the cell membrane after isolating a cell-attached patch. The signal to noise ratio is usually sufficiently great that a larger recording bandwidth may be used. However, the limitations of single electrode point clamping remain −− namely uncertainty of spatial and/or temporal control, and series resistance problems.

In this paper some aspects of the electrical and chemical-metabolic regulation of Ca channels that we have worked on will be dealt with. Since virtually nothing is known about the structure of the Ca channel the aim has been to study those properties important for cellular function. Eventually of course structural information will have to be correlated with these functional observations. The results were obtained in a variety of cell types from a variety of species, e.g. snail neurons, rat or guinea pig myocytes, rat PC-12 and chick dorsal root ganglion cells (13-17), and are quite generalizable.

III. ELECTRICAL REGULATION OF Ca CHANNELS

Ca channels are activated by depolarization and during a sustained depolarizing step the activity rises and then falls by processes called activation and inactivation respectively. We shall deal with activation first. This process occurs after a delay and the kinetics for whole cell currents have been fitted by a first order process raised to powers ranging from second to fifth to account for the delay (18,19). The approach is taken from the model for Na channels (20) using the activation variable, m. The reaction for an m^2 model is

$$C_1 \underset{\beta_m}{\overset{2\alpha_m}{\rightleftharpoons}} C_2 \underset{2\beta_m}{\overset{\alpha_m}{\rightleftharpoons}} 0 \tag{1}$$

and

$$m = m_\infty - (m_\infty - m_0 e^{-t/\tau_m}) \tag{2}$$

describes the time course of the activation variable. Also,

$$\tau_m = (\alpha_m + \beta_m)^{-1} \tag{3}$$

This scheme predicts that relaxation of tail currents (see below) from a non-zero value of m_o to a zero value of m_∞ at the resting potential occurs along a monoexponential trajectory with time constant τ_m scaled according to the power used for m. Schemes of this sort can no longer be justified. Tail currents produced when the potential is stepped from a level that has activated all of the Ca channels to a level where the activation falls to zero, relax not with one but with two time constants (Fig. 1) (15,18,21,22).

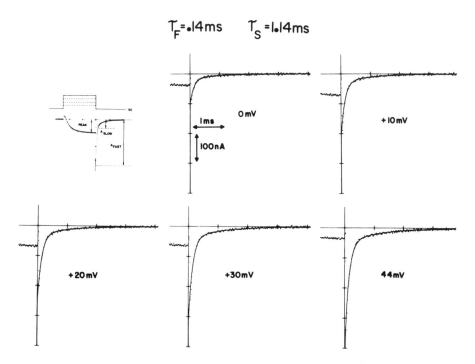

FIGURE 1. Turn-off of I_{Ca}. Ca tail currents were measured at −50 mV following activation to different potentials. The parameters were estimated using a non-linear least squares fitting routine (18,21) and points in the first 150 μsec were not considered in the error criteria. As described in (18,21), from an initial approximation the time constants did not appear to be a function of the pulse potential ($\tau_F = 0.14 \pm 0.01$ msec and $\tau_S = 1.14 \pm 0.15$ msec); the time constants were thus constrained to the mean values and the resulting curve fits are shown.

The fast time constant is about 150 μsec at 20°C and is only weakly voltage-dependent. The slow time constant is about 10 times larger than the first and is strongly voltage dependent. Hence literal H-H models are excluded and for the two time constant process of the tail currents, at least three states are required. Note that the deactivation of tail currents is the opposite sequence to activation. In activation the channels start in C_1 (Eq. 1) and proceed to 0. In deactivation the channels start in 0 and proceed to C_1.

The situation is even more complicated however. The two tail time constants cannot account for the delay in turn-on of whole cell currents. The turn-on requires at least two time constants but both are much larger than the fast tail time constants. Moreover cooling produces a marked slowing in rate of turn-on but has only a small effect on the tail current time constants (Fig. 2).

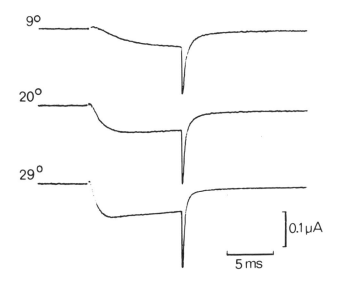

FIGURE 2. Effects of changes in temperature on activation of macroscopic current. Whole cell Ca currents were recorded from an isolated nerve cell body. The voltage step was to +20 mV and the return potential was −15 mV. The levels were attained within 60 sec. Each record was the average of 15 runs which have been corrected for linear leakage and capacitive currents, with the correction currents produced by an inverted pulse program. The uncorrected traces showed instantaneous rises to very large amplitudes with a subsequent time course similar to the deactivated records.

Finally the latencies to first opening for single channels, or waiting times, cannot be fitted by the rate constants
calculated for a three state model of activation (Fig. 3).

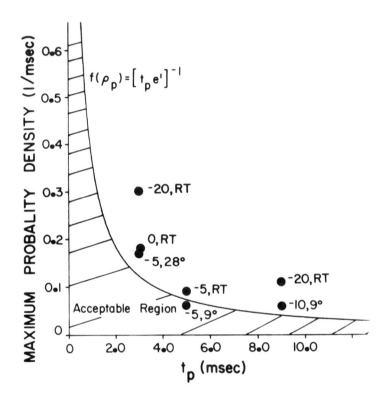

FIGURE 3. The smooth curve is the maximum allowable value
of the peak of the waiting time probability density plotted as
a function of t_p as obtained in Eq. 6 for a three-state model.
Measured values must lie in the "acceptable region" in order
for the data to be consistent with a three-state model. Data
obtaied under various conditions are plotted with the potential and temperature indicated. Note that all but one of the
data points lie outside this region, indicating an incon-
sistency with the model. For the following three-state
sequential model.

$$R \underset{k_{-1}}{\overset{k_{+1}}{\rightleftarrows}} A \underset{k_{-2}}{\overset{k_{+2}}{\rightleftarrows}} 0$$

the probability density function for the waiting time is given by

$$\omega(t) = \frac{\rho_1 \rho_2}{\rho_2 - \rho_1} e^{-\rho_1 t} - \frac{\rho_1 \rho_2}{\rho_2 - \rho_1} e^{-\rho_2 t} \qquad (4)$$

where

$$\rho_1, \rho_2 = 0.5 \ (k_{+1}+k_{-1}+k_{+2}) \pm [(k_{+1}+k_{-1}+k_{+2}) - 4k_{+1}k_{+2}]^{0.5}$$

The peak value of Eq. 4 as a function of time is found by setting the derivative to zero, solving for the time to peak, t_p, and reinserting the value into Eq. 4. After considerable rearrangement it is found that the maximum value of Eq. 4 is given by

$$\omega_{max} = \rho_1 e^{-t_p \rho_1} = \rho_2 e^{-t_p \rho_2} = f(\rho) \qquad (5)$$

Eq. 5 thus relates ω_{max}, t_p, and the two values. When $f(\rho)$ is plotted it is found to be a bell-shaped curve with a maximum. The maximum value of this curve occurs at ρ_p and is

$$f(\rho_p) = [t_p e^1]^{-1} \qquad (6)$$

Note that this equation yields the maximum admissible values for ω_{max} in Eq. 4.

Given the results to this point we have proposed a minimum four state diagram for activation,

$$C_1 \underset{k_{-1}}{\overset{k_{+1}}{\rightleftharpoons}} C_2 \underset{k_{-2}}{\overset{k_{+2}}{\rightleftharpoons}} C_3 \underset{k_{-3}}{\overset{k_{+3}}{\rightleftharpoons}} 0 \qquad (7)$$

It is the early forward transitions that control turn-on. Presumably these are quite voltage- and temperature-dependent.

We can make some further statements about the rate constants as well. The rate constant k_{ij} for the transition from i to j as a function of membrane potential is from absolute rate theory

$$k_{ij}(V) = Ae^{-U_{ij}(V)/kT} \tag{8}$$

where the constant A includes the transmission coefficient, T is temperature, k in the exponent is the Boltzmann constant and differs from the rate constant k_{ij}, and U_{ij} is the free energy difference that must be surmounted for the transition from i to j to occur. At lower depolarizations, inactivation is negligible and it can be ignored in the state diagram. Over this range neither potential nor temperature changes alter open time substantially. Hence k_{-3} (Eq. 7) which is the reciprocal of the open time must involve a very subtle molecular rearrangement. On the other hand, the sensitivity to temperature of the turn-on process suggests that k_{+1} or some earlier forward transition rate constant (recall that our model is a minimum one) have a high temperature coefficient and strong voltage-dependence. From the closed time distributions we plan to evaluate the rate constants in this scheme using the approach of Colquhuon and Hawkes (23), and compare their values at different temperatures and potentials.

Single channel recording provides further insight into how cooling slows the rate of activation and reduces peak currents (Fig. 4). For a 20 degree change in temperature unit conductance was reduced by about 30 percent with a Q_{10} of 1.5. Mean open times were unchanged and bursts and gaps within bursts appeared unaltered. However the rate of opening was reduced five fold with a Q_{10} of three. Hence the effects of cooling support our interpretation of the whole cell or macroscopic current results namely that an early transition among closed states has a large temperature coefficient.

Other interesting facts have emerged from the single channel measurements. As noted the unitary currents are due to about 3,000 Ca ions entering per average open time of 1 msec. The channel densities are estimated at about $1-10/\mu m^2$ for a wide range of cells assuming homogeneous distributions. However, it appears that these may differ from results of binding studies. For example the number of binding sites may be regulated by extracellular divalent cation concentration or species whereas the number of functional Ca channels is not. Moreover the high affinity dissociation constants for the dihydropyridine class of Ca antagonists used in the binding experiments usually differs from the IC_{50} of the functional measurements.

The Ca channels appear to have only two conductance states, open and closed. In many hundreds of recordings we have never observed any sub- or super-conductance states. The open times have simple exponential distributions and these findings are consistent with a single open state. The channels appear to behave independently. Whenever a patch contains two active channels the occurrence of simultaneous events can be predicted from the binomial theorem.

To this point we have paid no attention to the inactivation process. Figure 4 shows Ca currents averaged from single channel records rise and fall as do whole cell Ca currents. These results exclude the possibility of contamination by other currents. Neither amplitude nor mean open time were changed and the principal effect was a reduction in opening rate at longer times. Depletion or accumulation pro-

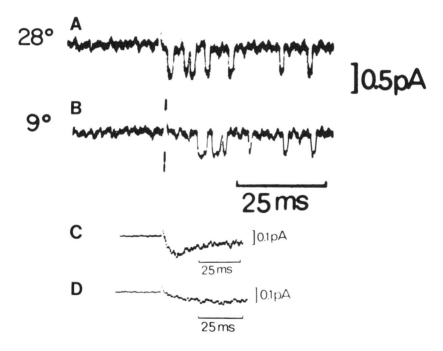

FIGURE 4. Effects of temperature on single Ca channels (A and B). Records are from the cell body of a snail neuron voltage clamped with two microelectrodes and patch clamped with the gigaseal method. Holding potential, V_H was −50 mV, command potentials V_e were zero mV and the onsets are shown by the artefacts in each record. Ca in patch pipette was 40 mM. Linear components of leakage and capacitance have been subtracted. The currents were summed from 68 samples in C and 72 samples in D. There were no failures in C and 15 in D.

cesses can be clearly excluded because the unitary amplitudes
were unchanged. Averaged single channel currents could be
scaled to whole cell currents which make a Ca-mediated
cytoplasmic process unlikely. In addition bursts have little
effect on subsequent average opening probabilities, a result
that would not be predicted by models in which inactivation is
produced exclusively by entering Ca ions reacting with the
channel (24,25). Standen and Stanfield (24,25) probably err
in their claim that tail currents are responsible for the fact
that h_∞ does not return to 1.0 when prepulses near E_{Ca} are
delivered. They modeled activation as an m^2 process but the
tail time constants are 10 times faster than predicted by this
scheme and cannot, as we have indicated, be attributed to an
m^2 process. Hence Ca entry during tails was grossly over-
estimated.

We turn now to a consideration of factors that affect Ca
channel activity which are not primarily related to changes in
membrane potential.

IV. NON-ELECTRICAL REGULATION OF Ca CHANNELS

There are several examples of chemicals modifying Ca
currents. The most important physiologically is the sympathetic neurotransmitter, norepinephrine, or NE, which acts
on heart cells to increase I_{Ca}. This is achieved probably in
two ways -- first by increasing the rate at which single channels open (26), and second by increasing the number of channels N available for activation (27).

Other agents which modulate Ca channel activity include
serotonin and GABA (28,29). It is not known whether these
agents act on non-voltage-dependent Ca channels or whether
action is mediated by voltage-dependent channels. More
recently Yatani et al. (30) have demonstrated a purinergic
receptor in snail neurons that is activated by nanomolar concentrations of ATP. Activation of the receptor in turn
increases the voltage-dependent Ca currents although it is not
known whether the number of channels or the elementary current
or both are affected.

Another way in which Ca channel activity is modulated is
by Ca ion itself. Changes in Ca_o act to change the gating of
the Ca channel via an action on surface charge (Fig. 5)(1).
Ca currents provide two measures of these effects. This is
because the maximum shift in gating occurs at concentrations
where the surface concentration according to surface charge
theory (1), is independent of the bulk concentration. Hence
gating shifts are largest when current-concentration curves
show saturation. The figure shows the effects of Mg on Ca

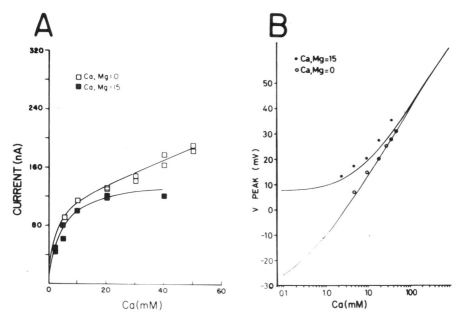

FIGURE 5. Effects of divalent cations on current-concentration relationships (A) and gating (B). Experiments were done on Helix neurons that were voltage clamped and internally perfused (1). V_H was -50 mV, V_C was +10 mV and Ca_O was 10 mM. The solid lines are the fits from the surface charge model using constant field assumptions for the instantaneous I-V relation. Saturation in the current-concentration curve is due to the fact that over these range of concentrations surface concentration changes very little when bulk cocentration is changed. Over this range the shifts in gating measured as the change in $V_{1/2}$ of the activation curve for I_{Ca}, are maximal. M_g ion by reducing surface charge, reduces surface concentration of Ca and hence Ca currents. It also results in large shifts in gating.

current amplitude and gating. The fits to surface charge theory (31) are very good.

An interesting addition to this story is the fact that it is not necessary to attribute a larger conductance in Ca channels to Ba ions. Differences between Ba and Ca in binding to surface charge can just as easily account for the results. Hence a lower affinity of Ba is associated with a higher surface concentration and gating at more negative potentials.

Intracellular Ca does not shift gating in an obvious way but this may be only because the intracellular concentrations are too low to affect surface charge. However large levels of

Ca_i in the micromolar range inactivate Ca channels (5,32,33).
The recovery from inactivation of Ca currents is clearly
influenced by Ca entry (5,32,33).   Agents which reduce Ca_i
such as EGTA and possibly ATP, speed the recovery process
(Fig. 6).

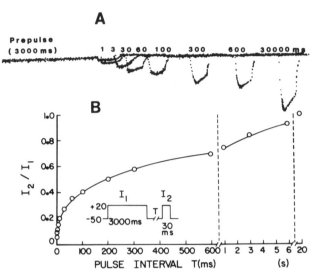

FIGURE 6.   Recovery of I_{Ca} following a 3 sec prepulse
which produced complete inactivation.
A.   Ca current records 1, 3, 30, 60, 100, 300, 600 and 30,000
msec following a 3 sec prepulse.   Note that the current at the
end of the prepulse is zero.   Recovery begins within 1.0 msec
and recovery current shows faster rates of inactivation as
their amplitude increases.
B.   Peak Ca current during the test depolarization (I_2) was
normalized by peak I_{Ca} during the immediately preceding con-
ditioning pulse (I_1).   There was complete inactivation of the
Ca current yet as noted, there was not delay visible in the
recovery curve.

     The recovery of Ca current occurs with two time constants
just as the onset of inactivation during a single pulse shows
two time constants.   Moreover the recovery process occurs
without any discernible delay .   The significance of this is
unclear since the onset of inactivation may show some delay.
A more complete model of Ca currents should therefore include
these two inactivation states.   Given the arguments against an
obligatory coupling of inactivation to activation and the evidence for voltage-dependent inactivation, a minimum state

diagram based upon present certainties and uncertainties might
be:

$$C_1 \underset{\longleftarrow}{\overset{\longrightarrow}{}} C_2 \underset{\longleftarrow}{\overset{\longrightarrow}{}} C_3 \underset{\longleftarrow}{\overset{\longrightarrow}{}} 0 \qquad (9)$$

with

$$I_1 \underset{\longleftarrow}{\overset{\longrightarrow}{}} I_2$$

V. SUMMARY

In this report I have related single channel and whole
cell measurements of Ca currents. It is clear that Ca channel
activity which regulates so many cell functions is in turn
regulated by membrane potential and certain chemicals
including calcium ion itself. There are at least six potential dependent conformations for the channel. The transition
rate constant from the open to the closed state is weakly
voltage- and temperature-dependent and one of the early forward transitions has a high temperature coefficient.

ACKNOWLEDGMEMT

It is a pleasure to acknowledge my collaboration with
Dieter Lux, Diana Kunze, and Dave Wilson.

REFERENCES

1. Wilson, D. L., Morimoto, K., Tsuda, Y., and Brown, A. M.,
    J. Membr. Biol. 72:117 (1983).
2. Lux, H. D., and Brown, A. M., J. Gen. Physiol. 83:727
    (1984).
3. Hagiwara, S., "Membrane Potential-Dependent Ion Channels
    in Cell Membrane" Raven Press, New York, 1983.
4. Fatt, P., and Katz, B., J. Physiol. 121:374 (1953).
5. Hagiwara, S., and Naka, I. -I., J. Gen. Physiol. 48:141
    (1964).
6. Hagiwara, S., Ozawa, S., and Sand, O., J. Gen. Physiol.
    65:617 (1975).
7. Kostyuk, P. G., and Krishtal, O. A., J. Physiol. 270:545
    (1977).

8. Akaike, N., Lee, K. S., and Brown, A. M., J. Gen. Physiol. 71:509 (1978).
9. Lee, K. S., Akaike, N., and Brown, A. M., J. Gen. Physiol. 71:489 (1978).
10. Takahashi, K., and Yoshii, M., J. Physiol. 315:515 (1981)
11. Akaike, N., Fishman, H. M., Lee, K. S., Moore, L. E., and Brown, A. M., Nature 274:379 (1978).
12. Krishtal, O. A., Pidoplichko, V. I., and Shakhovolov, Y. A., J. Physiol. 310:423 (1981).
13. Lux, H. D., and Nagy, K., Pflügers Arch. 391:252 (1981).
14. Reuter, H., Stevens, C. F., Tsien, R. W., and Yellen, G., Nature 297:501 (1982).
15. Fenwick, E. M., Marty, A., and Neher, E., J. Physiol. 331:577 (1982).
16. Brown, A. M., Camerer, H., Kunze, D. L., and Lux, H. D., Nature 299:156 (1982).
17. Hagiwara, S., and Ohmori, H., J. Physiol. 336:649 (1983).
18. Brown, A. M., Tsuda, Y., and Wilson, D. L., J. Physiol. 344:549 (1983).
19. Llinas, R., Steinberg, I. Z., and Walton, K., Biophys. J. 33:289 (1981).
20. Hodgkin, A. L., and Huxley, A. F., J. Physiol. 117:500 (1952).
21. Tsuda, Y., Wilson, D. L., and Brown, A. M., Biophys. J. 37:181a (1982).
22. Byerly, L., Bryant, C. P., and Stimers, J. R., J. Physiol. 348:187 (1984).
23. Colquhuon, D., and Hawkes, A. G., Proc. R. Soc. Lond. B. 211:205 (1981).
24. Standen, N. B., and Stanfield, P. R., Proc. R. Soc. Lond. B. 217:101 (1982)
25. Chad, J., Eckert, R., and Ewald, D., J. Physiol. 347:279 (1984).
26. Cachelin, A.M., and Reuter, H., Nature 301:569 (1983).
27. Bean, B. P., Norwicky, M.C., and Tsien, R.W., Nature 307:371 (1984).
28. Pellmar, T. C., and Carpenter, D. O., Nature 277:483 (1979).
29. Dunlap, K., and Fischbach, G.D., J. Physiol. 317:519 (1981).
30. Yatani, A., Tsuda, Y., Akaike, N., and Brown, A. M., Nature 296:169 (1982).
31. Stern, Z., Electrochemistry 30:508 (1924).
32. Tillotson, D., and Horn, R. Nature 273:312 (1978).
33. Yatani, A., Wilson, D. L., and Brown, A. M., Cell. Molec. Neurobiol. 3:381 (1984).

Ca CHANNEL IN THE GH₃ CELL

H. Ohmori

Department of Neurobiology
Brain Research Institute
Faculty of Medicine
University of Tokyo
Bunkyo-ku, Tokyo

I. INTRODUCTION

The clonal pituitary cell (GH_3) of rat generates action potentials (1,2), and it has been shown that both Na and Ca components exist in the action potential. Since the cell size is small enough for the application of the patch clamp technique to the whole cell in voltage clamp experiments, and the gating of the Ca channel is slow enough for accurate measurements, the gating kinetics of the GH_3 Ca channel were studied analyzing the whole cell currents and the single channel currents (3,4).

II. MACROSCOPIC PROPERTIES OF Ca CHANNELS

The procedure of the whole cell clamp and the surface patch clamp has been described elsewhere (3,4). When the concentration of the external Ca ion was increased from the normal value of 2.5 mM in Na-free TEA medium, an inward current with slow activation kinetics was observed (Fig. 1A). These kinetics become faster as the membrane is depolarized. Similar activation kinetics were observed when Ca was replaced with either Sr or Ba. The permeability sequence is $Ba > Sr > Ca$.

The inward current carried by Ca showed time dependent decay during 200 msec command pulse (Fig. 1A). This decay is not due to the inactivation of the Ca channel, but is due to

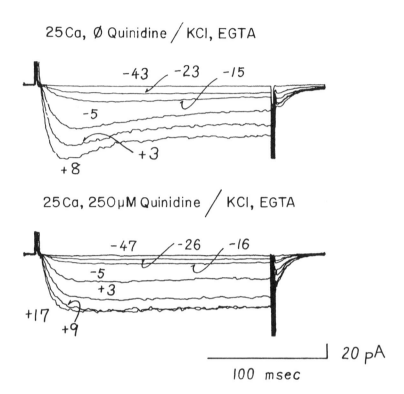

25 Ca, Ø Quinidine / KCl, EGTA

25 Ca, 250 μM Quinidine / KCl, EGTA

20 pA

100 msec

FIGURE 1. Whole cell Ca channel currents. When membrane potential was positively changed by a command pulse from −60 mV to the level indicated in the figure, inward currents with slow activation kinetics were observed. The decay observed in traces in A disappeared after bath application of 250 μM quinidine. The kinetics without decay is therefore the gating kinetics of the GH₃ Ca channel (traces in B). Even without using quinidine, typical kinetics were observed in Ba saline in which most experiments were performed (Hagiwara 1983 (5), with permission).

the activation of a Ca activated K conductance on the basis of the following: (i) In the Ba solution there is no decay in the current (Fig. 2A). (ii) When the isotonic CsCl solution was used in a patch electrode with a relatively large tip diameter (1-2 μm) to facilitate the exchange of the CsCl with the intracellular medium, the decay was eliminated even in Ca-containing external solution. (iii) Small quantities (100-200 μM) of either quinine or quinidine in the extracellular medium effectively eliminated the decay in Ca currents (Fig. 1B). Quinine and quinidine are known to block Ca activated K con-

ductance in several preparations.   Therefore, the kinetics
without decay seem to be the typical kinetics of the GH₃ Ca
channel, and it was concluded that the activation follows the
m² kinetics of the Hodgkin-Huxley model.   This conclusion was
derived from (i) a curve fitting procedure to the rising phase
of the Ba current, and (ii) a comparison of time constant of
the activation and the tail current after a step change of the
membrane potential from a fixed prepulse level to various test
potentials.   Although second order kinetics have been proposed
for the activation of some Ca channels (6), the Hodgkin-Huxley
model of cooperative first order kinetics has been adopted
here for simplicity of analysis.

III. STOCHASTIC NATURE OF Ca CHANNELS

Ionic currents are supposed to consist of a large number
of individual currents through single ionic channels distributed throughout the membrane.   This idea has been examined in
the Na channel, K channel and in the ACh receptor channel
first by noise analysis and more recently by single channel
recording.   Before applying the patch clamp technique to
obtain single Ca channel currents, a noise analysis was done
to estimate the size of the unitary current, density of the
channel, and temporal properties of the gating, all the information useful in the detection of these currents.

Assuming that the Ca channel has two conductance states,
open and closed, the mean current and the variance would be
expressed on the basis of the binomial distribution, where p
is the channel open probability, i is the single channel
current and N is the number of channels, as

$$I = N \ i \ p \qquad\qquad (1)$$

$$\sigma^2 = N \ i^2 \ p \ (1-p) \qquad\qquad (2)$$

Taking the ratio between the average current (I) and the
variance (σ^2) at each time point, the following equation can
be derived:

$$\sigma^2/I = i \ (1-p) = i - I/N \qquad\qquad (3)$$

Since the single channel current (i) and the number of channels (N) are considered to be time independent parameters, we
can expect a linear relation between the ratio (σ^2/I) and the
mean current (I).   From the plot of this ratio against the
average current at the corresponding time, we can estimate the
single channel current i as the y-intercept and the number

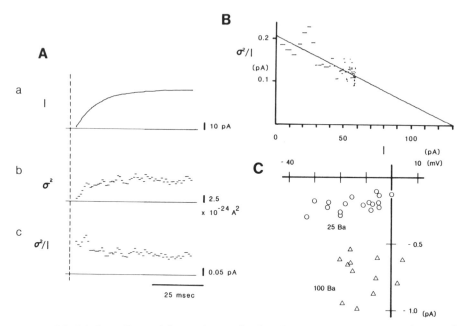

FIGURE 2. Ensemble noise of the Ba current measured at −6
mV. A, ensemble average ($\underline{I}$), variance (σ^2) and the ratio
($\sigma^2/\underline{I}$) between the two. Note that the ensemble average is
plotted as upward negative. B, the ratio ($\sigma^2/\underline{I}$) was plotted
against average current ($\underline{I}$) at the corresponding time. The $\underline{y}$-
intercept indicates single channel current amplitude as −0.2
pA, and the slope indicates the number of Ca channels as 650
per cell. C, estimated values of single Ba current through a
Ca channel were plotted against membrane potential in 25 mM Ba
and in 100 mM Ba saline (Hagiwara and Ohmori 1982 (3), with
permission).

of channels $\underline{N}$ from the reciprocal of the slope (Fig. 2A, B).
The estimate of the single channel Ba current was about −0.2
pA in the 25 mM Ba solution and about −0.6 pA in the 100 mM Ba
solution, both at 0 mV membrane potential (Fig. 2C). The
number of Ca channels was from 400 to 1,000 per cell. Since
the cell diameter was approximately 14 μm, channel density was
probably less than one per μm^2.

The microscopic kinetic properties of the Ca channel can
be understood through measurement of the steady state noise
spectrum (Fig. 3). The spectrum agrees well with the m^2
gating kinetics. However, closer inspection sometimes
revealed a systematic deviation of power at the higher frequency region. The existence of the higher frequency component in the spectrum is inconsistent with the m^2 type gating

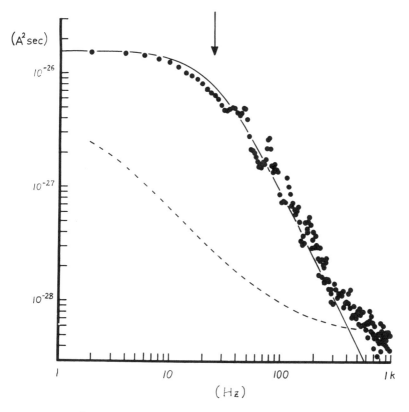

FIGURE 3. Power density spectrum of the steady state Ba current fluctuation. The smooth curve indicates a single Lorentzian spectrum with the cut off frequency indicated by the arrow. The broken line indicates level of the background noise. The measured spectrum was fitted well by the single Lorentzian spectrum. However, the spectrum deviated from the curve downward at low frequencies and upwards at high frequencies suggesting a more complex origin of the fluctuation than the m^2 kinetics (Hagiwara and Ohmori 1982 (3), with permission).

kinetics, and indicates the existence of a much faster kinetics than the m^2 process. The m^2 process predicts a double Lorentzian spectrum, but the difference of cut-off frequencies is a factor of two, which is practically impossible to detect in the power density spectrum. To resolve the contradiction between the macroscopic observation of the m^2 kinetics and the microscopic indication of the existence of much faster kinetics, a recording was made from a single Ca channel from a cell attached patch.

IV. SINGLE Ca CHANNEL CURRENT

When a step depolarizing voltage was applied to the patch
electrode, pulse-like events were visible (Fig. 4). They were
identified as Ba currents through a single Ca channel on the

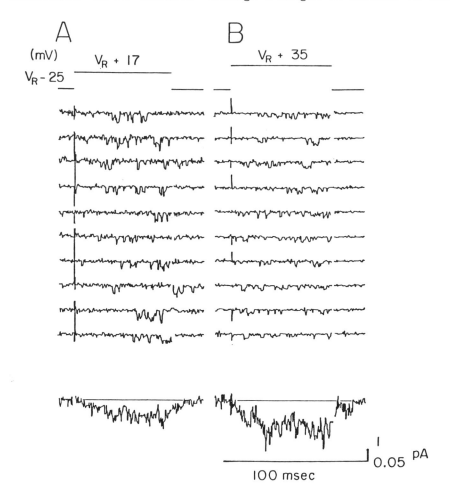

FIGURE 4. Single Ca channel currents recorded from a cell
attached patch membrane. V_R -10 mV in the present experimental condition: 25 MnCl$_2$, 1 MgCl$_2$, 125 TEA-Cl, 25 glucose,
2.5 quinidine, 10 HEPES-Na, in mM and pH 7.4.   Pipette was
filled with 100 mM Ba saline anticipating larger single channel currents than in the case of 100 mM Ca saline.   Bottom
traces were ensemble averages of single channel current traces
(Hagiwara and Ohmori 1983 (4), with permission).

basis of the following: (i) The time course of the activation of the average current became faster in response to a more positive voltage step. (ii) There was no inactivation of the

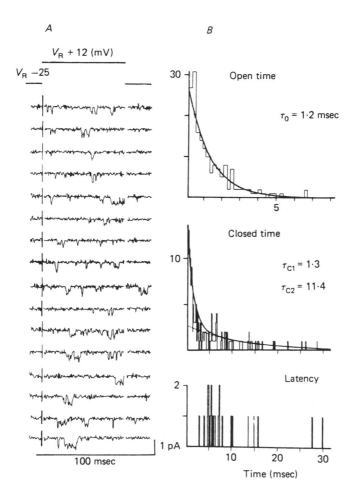

FIGURE 5. Single channel currents (A), and open time, closed time and latency histograms calculated from these currents (B). Open time histogram: an exponential curve (time constant of 1.2 msec) which gives the best fit to the histogram was visually determined and is illustrated by a continuous line. Closed time histogram: the continuous line was obtained by curve fitting using the sum of two exponential functions with time constants of 1.3 msec and 11.4 msec. Latency histogram: the major peak is found at around 5-6 msec, suggesting the presence of the rising phase (n=24) (Hagiwara and Ohmori 1983 (4), with permission).

current, at least in this 70 msec period. (iii) The amplitude
of the average current became larger at relatively depolarized
potential. (iv) The amplitude of each pulse like event became
smaller as the membrane was depolarized.

The open time, closed time and latency (the time of first
opening after start of the voltage pulse) were measured from
each single channel current trace (Fig. 5). The open time
histogram showed a single exponential decay with a time
constant of approximately 1 msec. The closed time histogram
clearly indicated more than a single exponential component.
The histogram was fitted with two exponential functions with
time constants of approximately 1 msec and a much larger
value. The latency histogram seemed to show peak events with
a certain delay after the start of the voltage pulse.

No potential dependence was detected in either the mean
open time or the shorter time constant of the closed time
histogram. The longer time constant of the closed time

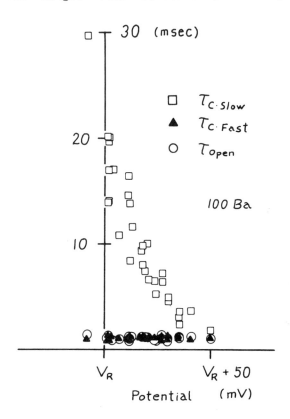

FIGURE 6. Time constants measured in the histograms were
plotted against the membrane potential. V_R -10 mV (Hagiwara
and Ohmori 1983 (4), with permission).

histogram clearly showed potential dependence, with a tendency
and absolute value close to the expectation from the m^2 gating
kinetics (Fig. 6). The latency histogrom showed potential
dependence similar to that of the longer time constant of the
closed time histogram (4). The feature of the open time
histogram is totally inconsistent with the gating kinetics of
the Hodgkin-Huxley model. What we can conceive from these
results is the existence of two unrelated gating kinetics:
one is slow and may be analogous to the m^2 kinetics of the
Hodgkin-Huxley model and the other is a very fast flickering
kinetics. The potential dependence of the latter remains
uncertain. Although no clear potential dependence was
detected in the fast flickering kinetics, a fast decaying tail
current was frequently observed in the other preparations
(6-8), which may indicate some sort of potential dependence of
the fast flickering kinetics in a more negative range of
membrane potential than that we used.

V. A MODEL FOR THE Ca CHANNEL GATING

A proposed model of the gating kinetics is shown in Fig.
7. We think it easy to explain our results with two independent gates: a potential dependent slow gate and a relatively
potential independent fast flickering gate. The horizontal
kinetic pathway is the slow potential dependent gating process
and the vertical pathway is the fast flickering kinetics. If
the fact of the fast tail current is true even in the GH$_3$
cell, most channels would be in state C_1^* at the resting
potential, and at depolarized potentials channels would
flicker between O and C*. The fast tail current would be
generated by the step from O to C*, and the slow tail current
by the closing process from O to C_2. From this gating scheme
we can understand the single exponential decay in the open
time histogram, and the multiple exponential decay in the
closed time histogram. Because of the limited number of
events, it is quite possible that we could not have detected
more than two exponential processes in the closed time
histogram. For the same reason we might have missed some sort
of potential dependence in both the open time histogram and
the fast decaying portion of the closed time histogram.
We prefer the above gating model to linear sequential
models, although the sequential model has an advantage at
least in the aspect that the histogram pattern can be
expected, quantitatively. Our results might be explained by
one of the following sequential models.

$$C_1 \xrightleftharpoons[b]{f} C_2^* \xrightleftharpoons[k_{-1}]{k_1} 0 \qquad (4)$$

$$C_1 \xrightleftharpoons[b_1]{f_1} C_2 \xrightleftharpoons[b_2]{f_2} 0 \xrightleftharpoons[k_{-1}]{k_1} C_3^* \qquad (5)$$

In either model the steps between 0 and C* are supposed to be very fast and will be seen as the fast flickering kinetics in a single channel recording. In scheme (4), we can expect a strictly potential independent process from the open time histogram by assuming k_{-1} as potential independent. However, the fast decaying process of the closed time histogram would become potential dependent to the same extent as the slow decaying process of the same histogram. In gating scheme (5), we expect the fast decaying component of the closed time histogram to be potential independent and open time histogram potential independent effectively by setting the values k_1 and k_{-1} substantially larger than the other rate constants. However, when the membrane potential is returned to the resting potential a significant number of the Ca channels must be in the closed state C_3^*; the number is proportional to the

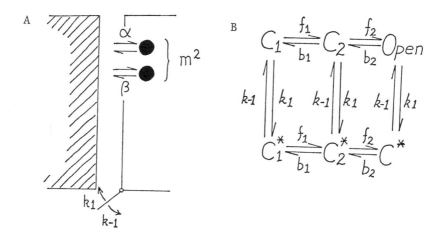

FIGURE 7. A model for the gating kinetics of the GH3 Ca channel. A, the gate indicated by a pair of filled circles is assumed as potential dependent slow kinetics, while that indicated by a rod is assumed as potential independent fast kinetics. B, the gating scheme derived from the model in A (Ohmori and Hagiwara 1983 (9), with permission).

ratio of $k_1/(k_1+b_2)$. The number of Ca channels in state C_3^* at the resting state would be much larger than those channels in the other closed states, if we assume the existence of the fast tail current in the GH_3 Ca channel; this assumption implies that $k_1 \gg k_{-1}$ at the negative membrane potentials. Since there is no possibility for the channel in C_3^* to return to the other closed states without passing through the open state, a significant portion of the Ca channel must open with very fast kinetics with the time constant of approximately 500 μsec macroscopically in response to the succeeding voltage pulse, and in the latency histogram we should have noticed a fast decaying process with a time constant similar to the fast component in the closed time histogram. Because of the presence of the capacitative transient a period close to 2 msec after the step voltage change may not be reliable in the present records. However, we were able to detect at least the tail of the fast decaying process in the latency histogram. The absence of such a tail in our single channel measurements and the absence of a very fast rising process in the macroscopic kinetics implies the existence of a pathway between closed state C_3^* and the other closed states. The model shown in Fig. 7 thus seems most reasonable and realistic given our present knowledge of Ca channel gating. Similar fast flickering kinetics has been observed in the Ca channel of other preparations (6,10,11) and also in the K channel (12) and in the Ca activated K channel (13).

REFERENCES

1. Kidokoro, Y., Nature, Lond. 258:741 (1975).
2. Biales, B., Dichter, M. A., and Tischler, A., Nature, Lond. 267:172 (1977).
3. Hagiwara, S., and Ohmori, H., J. Physiol., Lond. 331:231 (1982).
4. Hagiwara, S., and Ohmori, H., J. Physiol., Lond. 336:649 (1983).
5. Hagiwara, S. "Membrane Potential-dependent Ion Channels in Cell Membrane", Raven Press, New York, 1983.
6. Fenwick, E. M., Marty, A., and Neher, E., J. Physiol., Lond. 331:599 (1982).
7. Tsuda, Y., Wilson, D. L., and Brown, A. M., Biophys. J. 37:181a (1982).
8. Byerly, L., and Hagiwara, S., J. Physiol., Lond. 322:503 (1982).
9. Ohmori, H., and Hagiwara, S., in "The Physiology of Excitable Cells" (A. D. Grinnell, and W. J. Moody, Jr., eds.), p. 13. Alan R. Liss Inc., New York, 1983.

10. Lux, H. D., and Nagy, K., Pflügers Arch. 391:252 (1981).
11. Ohmori, H., J. Physiol., Lond. 350:561 (1984).
12. Conti, F., and Neher, E., Nature, Lond. 285:140 (1980).
13. Marty, A., Nature, Lond. 291:497 (1981).

ION CHANNELS ACTIVATED BY CALCIUM[1]

Makoto Endo

Department of Pharmacology
Faculty of Medicine
University of Tokyo
Bunkyo-ku, Tokyo

I. ION CHANNELS IN THE PLASMA MEMBRANE ACTIVATED BY Ca^{2+} ION

An increase in intracellular Ca^{2+} ion concentration in response to various stimuli to cells not only triggers a variety of biochemical reactions in the cells, as discussed in several chapters of this book, but also opens certain kinds of ion channels in cellular and intracellular membranes and thus regulates ion transport across these membranes. At least three such kinds of ion channels activated by Ca^{2+} ion are known at present. Two of them are channels in the plasma membrane and their activation probably contributes to regulate excitability of the cell. Only a brief description of these channels will be given, since the author has not yet studied them personally.

A. Ca-activated K Channel

Until the 1960s, the known mechanisms of control of passive ion transport across the cell membrane were either electrical control by membrane potential or a chemical one by neurotransmitters. In the early 1970s, Meech found a dif-

---

[1]This work was supported in part by Grants from Ministry of Education, Science and Culture, Japan and Ministry of Health and Welfare, Japan.

CALCIUM REGULATION
IN BIOLOGICAL SYSTEMS

197

ferent type of chemical control system; the injection of Ca^{2+} ion into molluscan nerve cells was shown to activate the K conductance of their plasma membrane (1). Since then, many studies (see ref. 2) including single channel studies with a recently developed patch clamp technique (3-6) have been made on this system in a wide variety of excitable cells. Thus, it is now quite well established that Ca^{2+} ion, acting on the plasma membrane from its protoplasmic side, opens a kind of ion channel which specifically allows K^+ ions to pass. Patch clamp studies revealed that an increase in intracellular Ca^{2+} ion concentration increased both the frequency and effective duration of channel openings, with first to third power relationship depending on cell species, but did not greatly alter the single channel conductance in the open state at least at lower Ca^{2+} ion concentrations (3,6). A submicromolar concentration of Ca^{2+} ion was usually effective, which suggests physiological involvement of this system (5,6). In this Ca-activated K channel, Ca^{2+} ion is not necessarily the only regulating factor, and the channel openings may also be dependent on membrane potential (3,6).

Intracellular Ca^{2+} ion concentration in nerve cells increases during excitation under a physiological condition as a result of the opening of a voltage-dependent Ca channel that are the subject of the chapters by Drs. Brown and Ohmori. This in turn, opens the Ca^{2+}-activated K channel, which tends to keep membrane potential near K equilibrium potential and hence to suppress the excitability. Thus, this system constitutes a negative feedback loop and appears to regulate the repetitive activity of nerve cells: if the more Ca^{2+}-activated K channels are open, they will exert an effect leading to a reduction of repetitive activity (2).

B. A Non-selective Cation Channel Activated by Ca^{2+} Ion

A different kind of ion channel in cardiac cell membrane is also shown to be activated by Ca^{2+} ion (7,8). Ion channels, probably of this type, in cardiac and neuroblastoma cells have been studied by patch champ technique as well (9,10). In this channel, Ca^{2+} ion also increases the probability of opening without altering the single channel conductance in the open state. This channel has several characteristics different from those of Ca^{2+}-activated K channels. It is permeable to alkali metal ions in a rather non-specific manner although not so unspecific as to allow passage of Ca^{2+} ion and anions (8-10). As a result, the opening of this channel causes depolarization in contrast to the hyperpolarization produced by the activation of Ca^{2+}-activated K channels, because Na permeability is more strongly increased than K permeability in this case. The opening of this channel is not appreciably dependent on membrane potential (9,10). A higher concentration of Ca^{2+} ion is required for activation of this channel than for the Ca^{2+}-activated K channel (9).

The physiological significance of this ion channel is not clear at present, but it may provide a background current required for pacemaker activity in cardiac cells (7-9). In a pathological state where the intracellular Ca^{2+} ion concentration is abnormally raised as in cardiac glycoside intoxication, it probably contributes to the resulting arrhythmia (7-9).

II. Ca-INDUCED RELEASE OF Ca FROM THE
SARCOPLASMIC RETICULUM

In the membrane of the sarcoplasmic reticulum (SR), there appears to be still another kind of ion channel activated by Ca. First known as a phenomenon called "Ca-induced Ca release" from the SR of skinned skeletal muscle fibers, this was found at about the same time independently by two groups in late 1960s, by Ford and Podolsky at NIH (11) and by us in Tokyo (12).

The properties of Ca-induced Ca release as studied in our laboratory using the SR of skinned muscle fibers will first be summarized. Since in the SR membrane a powerful Ca accumulating activity by Ca-Mg-ATPase or Ca pump ATPase is also present, Ca^{2+} ion applied to stimulate Ca-induced Ca release simultaneously stimulates the Ca pump, and as a result one can see only the net result of the two processes, stimulated Ca release and uptake. In order to examine only Ca-induced Ca release, Ca stimulation was therefore given in the absence of ATP to eliminate the Ca pump activity. Briefly, the experimental procedures used were as follows (13,14). After depleting Ca from the SR of a skinned fiber, a fixed amount of Ca was loaded to the SR. ATP in the environmental medium was then removed and various concentrations of Ca^{2+} ion were applied for various periods of time. The Ca^{2+} ion was then completely washed away, and the amount of Ca remaining in the SR was determined. The determination was made in a reversible manner utilizing a high concentration of caffeine to discharge all the Ca present in the SR, and the amount of Ca released was biologically assayed by the resulting contractile response of the skinned fiber itself. The difference in the remaining Ca with and without Ca^{2+} ion treatment in the absence of ATP was taken as the amount of Ca released by the Ca^{2+} ion treatment.

Figure 1 shows the relation between the amount of remaining Ca in the SR after the Ca^{2+} ion treatment and the duration of the treatment of the SR to which a fixed amount of Ca had been preloaded. When the Ca^{2+} ion concentration was low, the remaining Ca slowly decreased with time, indicating that Ca permeability of the SR membrane under this condition is very low. However, with an increase in the Ca^{2+} ion concentration, the remaining Ca decreased more and more rapidly (13). Thus, Ca^{2+} ion certainly induces Ca release.

The dependence of the initial rate of decrease in the remaining Ca, i.e., the rate of Ca release, on Ca^{2+} ion concentration differs among animal species, but it has the

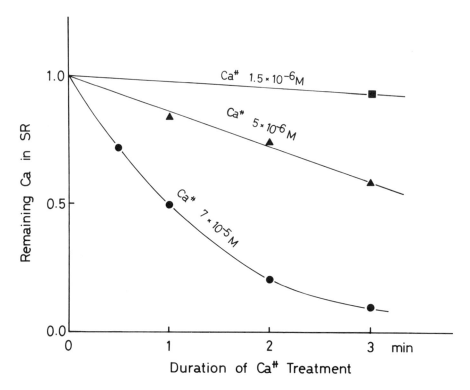

FIGURE 1. Time course of Ca release induced by Ca^{2+} ion in a skinned fiber of <u>Xenopus</u> skeletal muscle. After a fixed amount of Ca was loaded to the SR of the skinned fiber, ATP in the medium was removed and Ca ions were applied in the concentrations indicated in the figure for the period expressed on the abscissa. The Ca ions were then washed away, ATP was reintroduced and the amount of Ca remaining in the SR was determined by caffeine method (13) and plotted on the ordinate as value relative to that without the Ca treatment.

general form shown in Fig. 2 (13). Below a certain level of
Ca^{2+} ion concentration, the rate of Ca release was practically
independent of the Ca^{2+} ion concentration (not shown in Fig.
2), but above about 10^{-6} M in the example in Fig. 2, the rate
of Ca release started increasing. At the foot of the rising
phase, the Ca release rate was approximately proportional to
the square of Ca^{2+} ion concentration. With further increase
in Ca^{2+} ion concentration, the rate of Ca release tended to
saturate first and then to decrease. The falling phase may be
produced by the following two factors: (i) with higher Ca^{2+}
ion concentrations, the equilibrium point is closer to the
loading level and hence the driving force of Ca release is
less. (ii) Ca^{2+} ion itself may block the Ca channel, since
all the other divalent cations tested so far also decreased
the rate of Ca release at millimolar concentrations (13).

    Adenine nucleotides (15,16) and xanthine derivatives (17)
strongly enhance Ca-induced Ca release. The mode of action of
these two types of purine derivatives, however, is different.

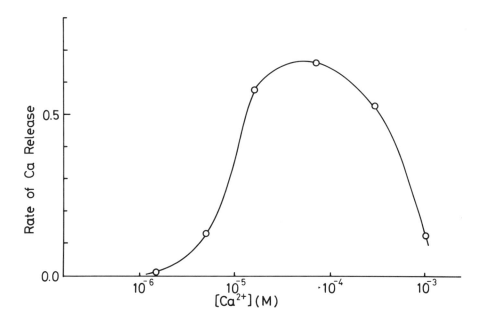

    FIGURE 2. The dependence of the rate of Ca release on
Ca^{2+} ion concentration. The initial rate of Ca release was
determined by experiments of the type depicted in Fig. 1, and
plotted against Ca^{2+} ion concentration. Ordinate is in units
of a reciprocal of the time required to reduce the amount of
Ca to zero, should the initial rate of release have continued
to the end. From ref. 13.

As shown in Fig. 3, adenine nucleotides increase the rate of Ca release without appreciably altering its Ca^{2+} ion concentration dependence (13). The effect of ATP is different from that of AMP shown in Fig. 3 in that ATP also increases the rate of Ca release in the Ca^{2+} ion concentration-independent region at lower levels of Ca^{2+} (see ref. 25). Among adenine nucleotides, ATP is the strongest in increasing Ca release rate, but this effect is qualitatively shared by all adenine compounds so far tested, AMPOPCP, AMPCPOP, ADP, AMP, cyclic AMP, adenosine and adenine (16). Unlike the adenine compounds, xanthine derivatives shift the dependence of Ca release rate on Ca^{2+} ion concentration to a lower concentration range in addition to their effect of increasing the maximum rate of Ca release at optimum Ca^{2+} ion concentration as is also shown in Fig. 3 (13).

Some local anesthetics such as procaine and tetracaine inhibit Ca-induced Ca release (18,19), but others such as cocaine, lidocaine (S. Yagi, unpublished observation) and dibucaine do not (20). Dibucaine is shown rather to enhance

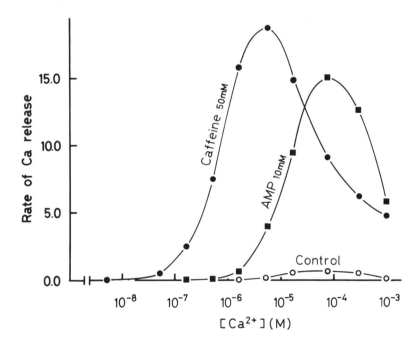

FIGURE 3. The effect of 10 mM AMP and 50 mM caffeine on Ca-induced Ca release. Rate of Ca release was determined as in Fig. 2. Potentiators were applied only during the Ca-induced Ca release in the absence of ATP. Cited from ref. 13 with a modification.

it. As shown in Fig. 4, procaine reduces the rate of Ca release without appreciably changing the Ca^{2+} ion concentration dependence (13). Mg^{2+} ion also inhibits Ca-induced Ca release, but unlike procaine, this ion appears to shift the dependence of Ca release rate on Ca^{2+} ion concentration to a higher concentration range (13), suggesting a competitive inhibition against the action of Ca^{2+} ion. However, since the inhibition by Mg^{2+} ion does not disappear even in the presence of a very high concentration of Ca^{2+} ion, inhibition of some mode other than competitive inhibition may also be present (Fig. 4).

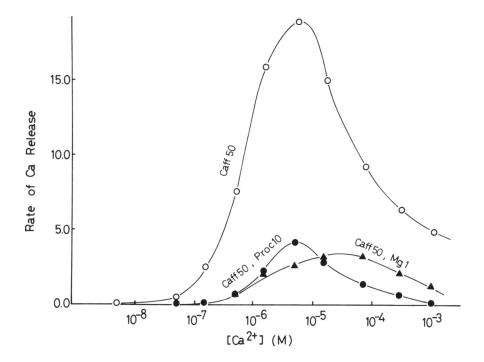

FIGURE 4. The effect of 10 mM procaine and 1 mM Mg^{2+} ion on Ca-induced Ca release. Experiments similar to those in Fig. 3. To make the inhibitory action clearer, these agents were applied in the condition where Ca-induced Ca release was enhanced by 50 mM caffeine. From ref. 13.

III. MECHANISM OF Ca-INDUCED Ca RELEASE

The main cause of Ca-induced Ca release is considered to be an increase in Ca permeability in the SR membrane. In other words, Ca^{2+} ion appears to open the "gate" of an "ion channel" through which Ca^{2+} ion can pass. Through this ion channel, Ca^{2+} ion rapidly flows out from the SR lumen under usual conditions because Ca^{2+} ion concentration in the lumen of the SR is much higher than that outside the SR. Supporting this idea, when Ca^{2+} ion concentration gradient is reversed, stimulation of Ca-induced Ca release by caffeine or other agents causes rapid inflow of Ca^{2+} ion into the SR lumen (21). This inflow appears to utilize the same mechanism as the Ca-induced Ca release, because it is inhibited by inhibitors of Ca-induced Ca release such as procaine and Mg^{2+} ion (21).

Ca^{2+} ions accumulated in the SR are mostly bound in the lumen of the SR, probably to the large capacity and low-affinity Ca-binding protein, calsequestrin (22). Therefore, a conceivable alternative mechanism of Ca release is liberation of bound Ca from calsequestrin, which increases free Ca^{2+} ion concentration in the SR lumen, and hence increases the rate of leakage or release of Ca^{2+} ion from there. However, whereas the complete liberation of Ca^{2+} ion from calsequestrin causes only about a 15-fold increase of Ca^{2+} ion concentration in the SR lumen, the release rate when Ca-induced Ca release is stimulated by a high concentration of caffeine is more than 1000-fold that of the leakage rate (21). This observation cannot be explained without assuming Ca permeability increase of the SR membrane during Ca-induced Ca release at least when stimulated by caffeine.

Because, as described in the previous section, the mechanism of Ca-induced Ca release involves interactions with Ca^{2+} ion and with ATP as does the mechanism of the Ca pump, it is conceivable that Ca-induced Ca release is another function of the Ca pump protein. Although it is clear that Ca-induced Ca release is not a reversal of the Ca pump (see ref. 23), the same protein might operate in two different manners through some unknown regulatory interconversion process, transporting Ca^{2+} ion into the SR actively at one time and causing Ca release from the SR lumen at another time (24). This possibility has been examined and excluded by the following facts (16). The ATP-binding site of the Ca-induced Ca release mechanism for the stimulating action has characteristics entirely different from ATP-binding sites of the Ca pump. The affinity of the former for ATP estimated from stimulation of Ca-induced Ca release is much higher than that of the enzymatic site of the Ca pump. It is also to be noted that for stimulation of Ca-induced Ca release by ATP, the hydrolysis of ATP is not required. Affinities of both sites for other nucleotides such as ITP, UTP, GTP and CTP as well as other adenine derivatives again differ greatly. The characteristics of the ATP-binding site of Ca-induced Ca release are also very different from another ATP-binding site of the Ca pump for the regulatory action.

Thus, the experiments so far done are consistent with the hypothesis that Ca^{2+} ion, acting on a component of the SR membrane other than the Ca pump, opens the "gate" of an "ion channel" through which Ca^{2+} ion can pass. Whether or not other kinds of ions can also pass the "channel" is not precisely known at present, but an experiment by Kasai and his colleagues suggests that cations as large as choline[+] ion can also pass this "channel" (25). Under normal circumstances, a concentration gradient across the SR membrane exists only for Ca^{2+} ions, and, therefore, net movement of only Ca^{2+} ions may occur as a result of the opening of this rather "unspecific channel".

IV. SIGNIFICANCE OF Ca-INDUCED Ca RELEASE

The "Ca-activated ion channel" in the SR membrane responsible for Ca-induced Ca release does not seem to play an important role in excitation-contraction coupling in skeletal muscle (23). If it does play, an inhibitor of Ca-induced Ca release should inhibit physiological contraction. However, as shown in Fig. 5, when procaine was applied to an intact single fiber of amphibian skeletal muscle, it strongly inhibited caffeine contracture which is due to an enhancement of Ca-induced Ca release (17), but did not inhibit at all, but even potentiated, K-induced contracture which, as in physiological contraction, is caused by depolarization of surface and T-tubule membrane (19). Similar results were obtained with adenine. Although adenine by itself enhances Ca-induced Ca release as does ATP, its efficacy is much smaller, and in the presence of ATP, therefore, adenine inhibits Ca-induced Ca release probably by displacing ATP from its site of enhancing action (26). Other actions of adenine on the SR or on the myofibrils are not prominent (26). Thus, adenine is a relatively specific inhibitor of Ca-induced Ca release in the presence of ATP. Adenine applied to an intact single muscle fiber inhibited caffeine contracture as expected, but it did not at all inhibit but even potentiated normal twitches (27). K-contractures were not inhibited either but were potentiated by adenine. Interestingly, if twitches were potentiated by a low concentration of caffeine, adenine exerted an inhibitory effect to reverse the potentiation by caffeine (27). If twitches were potentiated by other means, by replacing chloride in Ringer solution with nitrate or by adding Zn^{2+} ion, adenine again did not inhibit at all but potentiated them (27). These results clearly indicate that although the enhanced Ca-induced Ca release plays a major role in caffeine

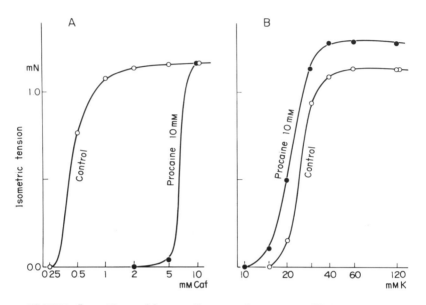

FIGURE 5. The effect of procaine on caffeine contracture (A) and on K contracture (B) of an intact single fiber.   A. Maximum tension developed by the fiber during 1 min application period of various concentrations of caffeine.   B. Maximum tension evoked by an application of various concentrations of K^+ ion.   Potassium-chloride product was kept constant, Tris and methanesulfonate being used as substituting ions.   Procaine was applied 30 sec before and was present throughout the application period of caffeine or K^+ ion.   From ref. 19.

contracture and a subsidiary role in caffeine potentiated twitches, if it is not enhanced, i.e., under normal condition, it does not play an important role in excitation-contraction coupling.

If the Ca-induced Ca release is pathologically enhanced in a hereditary disorder called malignant hyperthermia (28), it may play an essential role in the manifestation of the disease. Figure 6 shows dependences on Ca^{2+} ion concentration of the rate of Ca-induced Ca release from the SR of skeletal muscles of normal human beings and of a malignant hyperthermia patient with and without the influence of halothane (14). This drug shows an enhancing action on the Ca-induced Ca release similar to caffeine and is thought to be an inducing agent of malignant hyperthermia. It is clear that the Ca sensitivity of Ca-induced Ca release is higher and the maximum rate of Ca release at an optimal Ca^{2+} ion concentration greater in the patient's muscle than in normal one both in the

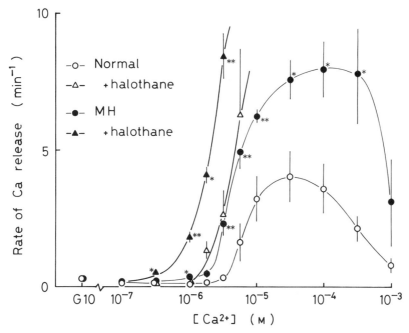

FIGURE 6.   Dependence of the rate of Ca release on the Ca^{2+} ion concentration in normal (open symbols) and malignant hyperthermia (closed symbols) fibers at 37°C in the presence of 1 mM Mg^{2+} ion.   Circles: without halothane.   Triangles: with 0.01% (v/v) halothane applied only during the Ca-induced Ca release.   From ref. 14.

absence and presence of halothane.   It was shown that this difference can explain the manifestation of the disease, i.e., under the influence of halothane only the patient's muscle may go into contracture while a normal one does not (14).

Thus in skeletal muscle, Ca-induced Ca release plays a role in inducing contractions only when it is enhanced pharmacologically or pathologically.

In cardiac muscle, Ca-induced Ca release appears to be evoked more easily than in skeletal muscle (29,30), and it has been proposed that physiological contraction of this kind of muscle may be caused by Ca release from the SR induced by the Ca ion itself that enters the cell in association with an action potential (29), although there is still no direct evidence to prove it.

In smooth muscles, Kuriyama and his colleagues (31) have shown that Ca-induced Ca release plays the major role in physiological contraction at least in pig coronary arteries. Whether or not this applies to other smooth muscles as well must soon be examined.

Some phenomena in cells other than muscle cells have been interpreted as a result of Ca-induced Ca release from the endoplasmic reticulum. (i) Repeated spontaneous transient hyperpolarization with an increase in K conductance was observed in the sympathetic ganglion cells of the bullfrog under the influence of caffeine (32). This may be the result of spontaneous Ca release from the endoplasmic reticulum due to Ca-induced Ca release enhanced by caffeine, which in turn opens the Ca-activated K channels. (ii) Propagated Ca release was demonstrated using aequorin in medaka eggs upon fertilization, and the most plausible explanation of the propagation is obviously the Ca-induced Ca release mechanism (33). (iii) Upon fertilization, the hamster egg shows transient, periodic hyperpolarizing responses due to a Ca-activated K conductance, which probably results from Ca-induced Ca release from intracellular stores (34). Although the first example mentioned above is a phenomenon in a pharmacologically modified state, the second and third examples appear to be those under a physiological condition. Thus, the Ca-induced Ca release mechanism might play a physiological role not in skeletal muscle cells where it was first discovered, but in certain kinds of cells where and when some additional amount of Ca is required.

REFERENCES

1. Meech, R. W., Comp. Biochem. Physiol. 42A:493 (1972).
2. Meech, R. W., Ann. Rev. Biophys. Bioeng. 7:1 (1978).
3. Marty, A., Nature 291:497 (1981).
4. Lux, H. D., Neher, E., and Marty, A., Pflugers Arch. 389:293 (1981).
5. Pallotta, B.S., Magleby, K. L., and Barrett, J. N., Nature 293:471 (1981).
6. Barrett, J. N., Magleby, K. L., and Pallotta, B. S., J. Physiol. 331:211 (1982).
7. Kass, R. W., Lederer, W. J., Tsien, R. W., and Weingart, R., J. Physiol. 281:187 (1978).
8. Kass, R. W., Tsien, R. W., and Weingart, R., J. Physiol. 281:209 (1978).
9. Colquhoun, D., Neher, E., Reuter, H., and Stevens, C. F., Nature 294:752 (1981).
10. Yellen, G., Nature 296:357 (1982).
11. Ford, L. E., and Podolsky, R. J., Science 167:58 (1970).
12. Endo, M., Tanaka, M., and Ogawa, Y., Nature 228:34 (1970).

13. Endo, M., in "The Mechanism of Gated Calcium Transport across Biological Membranes" (S. T. Ohnishi, and M. Endo, eds.), p. 257. Academic Press, New York, 1981.
14. Endo, M., Yagi, S., Ishizuka, T., Horiuti, K., Koga, Y., and Amaha, K., Biomed. Res. 4:83 (1983).
15. Endo, M., and Kitazawa, T., Proc. Japan Acad. 52:595 (1976).
20. Yagi, S., and Endo, M., Biomed. Res. 1:269 (1980).
21. Kitazawa, T., and Endo, M., Proc. Japan Acad. 52:599 (1976).
22. MacLennan, D. H., and Wong, P. T. S., Proc. Natl. Acad. Sci. USA 68:1231 (1971).
23. Endo, M., Physiol. Rev. 57:71 (1977).
24. Ogawa, Y., and Ebashi, S., J. Biochem. 80:1149 (1976).
25. Yamamoto, N., and Kasai, M., J. Biochem. 92:465 (1982).
26. Ishizuka, T., and Endo, M., Proc. Japan Acad. 59:93 (1983).
27. Ishizuka, T., Iijima, T., and Endo, M., Proc. Japan Acad. 59:97 (1983).
28. Denborough, H. A., and Lovell, R. R. H., Lancett II:45 (1960).
29. Fabiato, A., and Fabiato, F., J. Physiol. 249:469 (1975).
30. Endo, M., and Kitazawa, T., in "Biophysical Aspects of Cardiac Muscle" (M. Morad, ed.), p. 307. Academic Press, New York, 1978.
31. Itoh, T., Kuriyama, H., and Suzuki, H., J. Physiol. 321:513 (1981).
32. Kuba, K., and Nishi, S., J. Neurophysiol. 39:547 (1976).
33. Ridgway, E. B., Gilkey, J. C., and Jaffe, L. F., Proc. Natl. Acad. Sci. USA 74:623 (1977).
34. Igusa, Y., and Miyazaki, S., J. Physiol. 340:611 (1983).

PART III.
CALCIUM DEPENDENT PROTEASE

STRUCTURE AND FUNCTION OF Ca^{2+}-ACTIVATED PROTEASE

K. Suzuki

Department of Molecular Biology
Tokyo Metropolitan Institute of Medical Science
Bunkyo-ku, Tokyo

S. Kawashima
K. Imahori

Department of Biochemistry
Tokyo Metropolitan Institute of Gerontology
Itabashi-ku, Tokyo

I. INTRODUCTION

Ca^{2+}-activated (or dependent) protease (EC 3.4.22.17), a typical intracellular protease, exists ubiquitously in various organisms (reviews see 1-6). This protease was first extracted from rat brain in 1964 (7). It was also known at that time as a kinase activating factor (KAF) which activates phosphorylase b kinase in the presence of Ca^{2+} (8). Ca^{2+}-activated protease has recently received a great deal of attention with the recognition of the important role of Ca^{2+} in the control of cellular metabolism.

First, we shall define Ca^{2+}-activated protease as follows: "an intracellular thiol protease which requires Ca^{2+} for catalysis and is optimally active at a neutral pH region." CANP (Calcium-Activated Neutral Protease) is used here to denote this protease (9), although various names, e.g., calpain, KAF, and CAF (Calcium Activated Factor), have also been used. Two types of CANP, μCANP and mCANP, respectively activated at μM and mM orders of Ca^{2+}, have been identified in most tissues (4,10). They are also respectively called "types I and II", based on the order of elution from DEAE cellulose, or "low and high types", based on the concentration of Ca^{2+} required for

activity.   In this paper μM and mM orders refer to concentrations lower and higher than 0.1 mM, respectively,
because μCANP is active but mCANP is almost inactive at the
Ca^{2+} concentration.

The most striking characteristic of the intracellular protease is the strict control mechanism of enzyme activity.   If
the protease is always active in the cytosol, intracellular
proteins must be hydrolyzed at random and the cell will be
seriously damaged.   Thus the activity of intracellular
protease must be switched on only when it is required, and
switched off immediately after the protease has finished its
role.   The mechanism of regulation of enzyme activity is very
important for an understanding of the biological function of
intracellular protease.

TABLE I.   Properties of Purified μ and mCANPs

	μCANP	mCANP
Molecular weight	105 – 110K	105 – 120K
80K subunit	72 – 90K	74 – 80K
30K subunit	25 – 30K	25 – 31K
Ka value for Ca^{2+}	2 – 75 μM	0.2 – 0.8 mM
Optimum pH	6.8 – 8.0	7.0 – 8.0
Isoelectric pH	5.3 – 5.5	4.6 – 4.9
Heatstability (56°C, 20 min)	stable	unstable

Purified from

Skeletal muscle	rabbit[25,26] pig[27]	chicken[9], human[11] rabbit[12-14], pig[15]
Heart muscle	rat[16], pig[17]	rat[16], pig[17] bovine[18], monkey[19]
Other sources	rat kidney[21] bovine brain[22] human erythrocyte[28] human platelet[29] Ehrlich ascites tumor cell[30]	chicken gizzard[20] rat kidney[21] bovine brain[22] human platelet[23,24]

II. PROPERTIES OF CANP

CANP-like protease activity has been detected in various organisms (1-6). However, reports on its complete purification are relatively few. μ and mCANPs have been purified to complete or near homogeneity from the sources shown in Table I (9,11-30). Various properties of μ and mCANPs purified thus far are summarized in Table I. The overall features of both are quite similar. Their properties are: 1) Ca^{2+} is essential for activity, although the concentrations required are quite different; 2) CANP is a heterodimer composed of 80K (72K-90K) and 30K (25K-31K) subunits and shows the maximum activity at pH 6.8-8.0; 3) activity is inhibited by microbial thiol protease inhibitor like leupeptin, antipain and E64 and by thiol modifying reagents such as iodoacetic acid; 4) enzyme is inhibited specifically by endogenous protein inhibitor (calpastatin); 5) typical endopeptidase catalyzes limited proteolysis and no synthetic peptides thus far examined are hydrolyzed. Concentrations of Ca^{2+} for 50% activation (Ka) are 2-75 μM and 0.2-3 mM for μ and mCANPs, respectively. Thus the Ca^{2+} sensitivities of μ and mCANPs are clearly separated at 0.1 mM. Further, μCANP differs from mCANP with respect to heatstability and surface charge (25).

CANP hydrolyzes a limited number of proteins only to relatively large fragments, and hence only proteins such as casein and hemoglobin can be used for the assay. This makes it difficult to perform precise kinetic studies on CANP. Judging from the action of CANP on the insulin B-chain, peptide bonds susceptible to CANP are not specific to certain amino acid residues, but those involving hydrophobic amino acid residues are hydrolyzed (31). The tissue specificity of CANP is not known, but the contents of μ and mCANPs vary significantly. Figure 1 shows the amount of μ and mCANPs in various tissues of rat and chicken (32). Rat submandibular gland and kidney contain large amounts of both CANPs, whereas only mCANP was found in the chicken tissues examined.

III. PROPERTIES AND FUNCTION OF SUBUNITS OF CANP

The amino acid composition of the 80K and 30K subunits of μ and mCANPs are quite similar as shown in Fig. 2. Immunological analyses also indicate the similarity of 80K and 30K subunits of both CANPs (33). However, based on analyses of the peptide maps (33) and autolysis (34) it is concluded that the 80K subunits of μ and mCANPs, although similar, are clearly different and are probably the products of different genes,

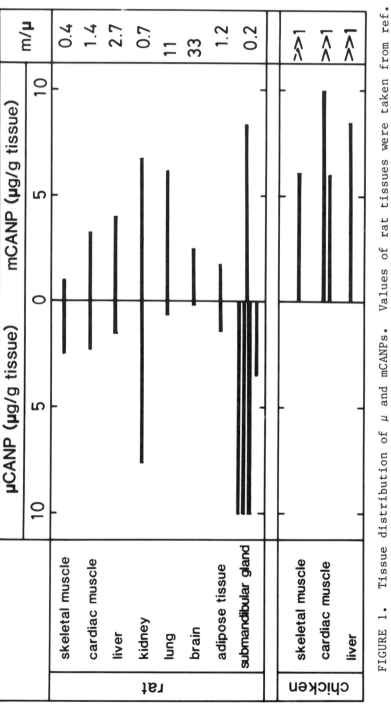

FIGURE 1. Tissue distribution of μ and mCANPs. Values of rat tissues were taken from ref. 32 and were recalculated assuming the specific activities of μ and mCANPs to be 287 and 642 units/mg, respectively (21). Values for chicken tissues are unpublished results estimated by enzyme linked immunosorbent assay.

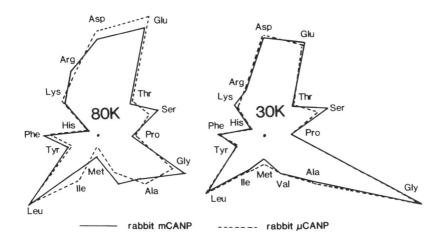

FIGURE 2.   Amino acid composition of the 80K and 30K subunits of rabbit muscle CANPs.

whereas the 30K subunits of both CANPs are identical or nearly
so.
      CANP without the 30K subunit has been isolated from
chicken and rabbit muscle (9,12). CANPs purified by chromatography on casein lack the 30K subunit (16,22), probably due
to autolysis during affinity chromatography in the presence of
Ca^{2+}. Studies on these CANPs indicate that various enzymatic
properties are indistinguishable, irrespective of the presence
of the 30K subunit. This clearly shows that the active site
is in the 80K subunit. In the presence of Ca^{2+}, iodoacetic
acid and E64 react with CANP very rapidly even at 0° and specifically label the cysteine residue in its active site
(35,36). The amino acid sequence around the cysteine residue
is shown in Fig. 3 (37). This is the first direct evidence
that CANP is a thiol protease. The sequence around the active
site cysteine resembles those of other thiol proteases, e.g.,
papain and cathepsin B. CANP differs clearly from these proteases with respect to molecular weight and requirement of
Ca^{2+} for activity. Nevertheless, the homologous active site
sequence indicates the same evolutionary origin. Presumably
CANP has enlarged during molecular evolution by acquiring
various specific regulatory functions.
      The role of the 30K subunit is not clear although its
similarity in μ and mCANPs suggests a specific common function. There are several possibilities. First, it may control
the activity of the 80K subunit, although the 30K subunit
probably dissociates in the presence of Ca^{2+} as is observed

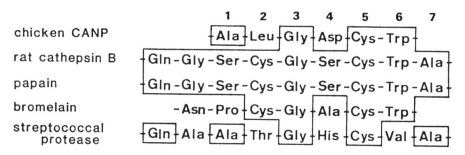

FIGURE 3.   Comparison of the amino acid sequence around the active site cysteine residue of chicken muscle mCANP with those of other thiol proteases.

with affinity chromatography on casein (16,22).   The 30K subunit does not affect known kinetic parameters of CANP, but some such unknown parameters could be affected.   Secondly, the 30K subunit may function as a kind of anchor in determining the location of CANP (80K subunit).   The conservation of amino acid composition may have some meaning.   This possibility is attractive but it has not been substantiated.   Thirdly, it may be produced by processing of a precursor of CANP and have no specific role.   Finally, the 30K subunit may protect the 80K subunit from degradation within the cell.

CANP dissociates into subunits in 8 M urea and the dissociated subunits can be separated by gel filtration or by chromatography on DEAE cellulose.   Reconstitution of CANP from the dissociated subunits occurs by removal of urea by dialysis. The 30K subunit is essential to regain the enzyme activity and full activity is obtained only when the equal amounts of the two subunits are added (13).   This is the only significance of the 30K subunit known at present but the meaning of this phenomenon is not yet clear.

IV. ACTIVATION OF CANP

The Ca^{2+} sensitivity of CANP suggests that μCANP is active but mCANP is not under a physiological concentration of Ca^{2+} (10^{-7}–10^{-6} M).   Since a fairly large amount of mCANP exists in cells as shown in Fig. 1, mCANP   must   play   some   role   under physiological conditions.   If mCANP plays any role in the cell, its Ca^{2+} sensitivity must be increased to have activity at a physiological Ca^{2+} concentration.   We found two methods of activation of   mCANP, by autolysis (38,39) and by an effector (Mn^{2+}) (40). In the presence of mM Ca^{2+}, limited autolysis of mCANP occurs. During autolysis the molecular weight of chicken mCANP changes from 80K to 79K and then to 60K (39). Ca^{2+} sensitivity is greatly increased by this autolysis. The Ka values of 79K and 60K species are both 30 μM, in contrast to 410 μM for the 80K species (mCANP). Therefore, we call these 79K and 60K species derived μCANPs I and II, respectively, to distinguish them from μCANP found in vivo (natural μCANP). The increase in Ca^{2+} sensitivity by autolysis is ascribed to hydrolysis of the 80K subunit. Change in subunit molecular weight during this activation is very small (25,34,39). Apparently only a small local conformation change is responsible for the significant change in Ca^{2+} sensitivity. This activation by autolysis is common to various CANPs (19,20,34). However, it is not clear whether or not this activation actually occurs in vivo. Derived μCANP is very similar to natural μCANP in various respects (38,39) but they are different molecules, because μ and mCANPs are different as discussed above (25,26,34). This type of activation is also observed with μCANP and the increase in Ca^{2+} sensitivity occurs (34).

mCANP is not active in mM Mn^{2+} or μM Ca^{2+} alone, but when mM Mn^{2+} and μM Ca^{2+} coexist, mCANP becomes active (19,40). Ca^{2+} sensitivity of mCANP changes in the presence of mM Mn^{2+} and the Ka value decreases from 410 μM to 40 μM in the case of chicken mCANP (40). This activation by Mn^{2+} will not occur in vivo because the required Mn^{2+} concentration (1-2 mM) is much higher than the intracellular concentration. However, the fact that Ca^{2+} sensitivity of mCANP can be controlled by an effector like Mn^{2+} is very important.

Intracellular Ca^{2+} concentration will not increase to the mM level under physiological conditions. Thus if Ca^{2+} sensitivity of mCANP does not change, mCANP becomes active only when an influx of extracellular Ca^{2+} occurs due to damage in the membrane permeability as is observed under some pathological conditions like muscular dystrophy. It is likely that the Ca^{2+} sensitivity of mCANP is increased in vivo by a certain mechanism as discussed here.

V. ROLE OF CALCIUM IONS

Figure 4 shows the titration of SH groups of native and modified CANPs (9,36,41). Carboxymethylation of the active site of mCANP reduces the number of SH groups which can be exposed to the solvent by conformation change induced by Ca^{2+}. In the case of native μCANP, no SH groups are exposed by addition of Ca^{2+}. Mn^{2+} and Ca^{2+} induce the same structural change

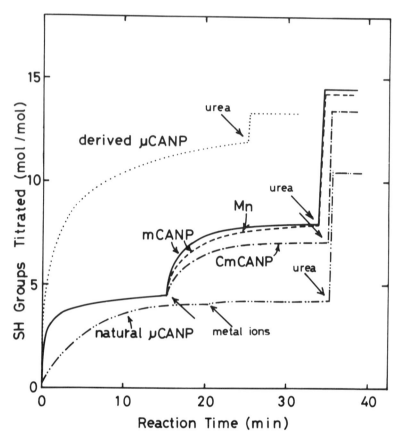

FIGURE 4.   Titration of SH groups of native and modified
CANPs. At the positions indicated, mM Ca^{2+} (or mM Mn^{2+} when
indicated) or 4 M urea was added.   Derived and carboxy-
methylated CANPs were prepared from chicken muscle mCANP.
Natural μ and mCANPs were isolated from rabbit and chicken
muscle, respectively.

in mCANP as judged by the titration curves in Fig. 4 and by
CD, UV and fluorescence measurements. Millimolar Ca^{2+} greatly
accelerates the rate of carboxymethylation of CANP.   If this
effect is ascribed to the exposure of the active site SH group
by conformation change, mM Mn^{2+} should have the same effect.
Nevertheless, mM Mn^{2+} does not accelerate carboxymethylation.
Simultaneous addition of mM Mn^{2+} and μM Ca^{2+} (0.1 mM),
however, greatly increases the rate of carboxymethylation of
mCANP as in mM Ca^{2+}.   These results show that Ca^{2+} not only
induces conformation change of CANP but activates the active
site SH group.

We have proposed a model for activation of mCANP mainly based on these results (Fig. 5) (41). mCANP has at least 2 Ca^{2+} binding sites. The dissociation constants of Ca^{2+} are of mM and μM orders, respectively, for the first and the second sites. The first site is exposed to the surface while the second site and the active site SH group are not accessible. When the Ca^{2+} concentration of the medium increases to the mM level, Ca^{2+} binds to the first site. This induces the conformation change of mCANP and exposes both the second site and the active site SH group to the surface. Since the dissociation constant of the second site is of the μM order and mM Ca^{2+} exists in the medium, Ca^{2+} binds to the second site immediately upon exposure and CANP becomes active. Mn^{2+} can bind to the first site in place of Ca^{2+} and induces the same conformation change. Therefore, in the presence of mM Mn^{2+} mCANP becomes active at μM Ca^{2+}. During autolysis the "cap" is removed by limited autolysis and the active site and the second binding site are always exposed (permanently open form or derived μCANP). Thus derived μCANP is active in the presence of μM Ca^{2+}. Titration of SH groups of natural and derived μCANPs (Fig. 4) suggests that the active site SH

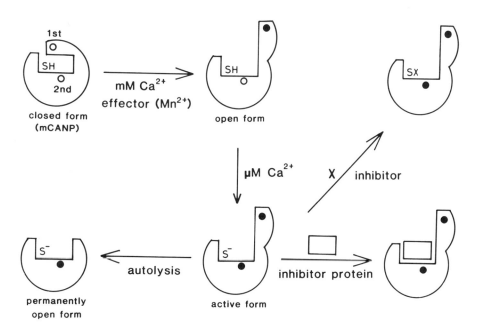

FIGURE 5. Activation of mCANP. o : vacant calcium binding sites. Filled symbols indicate the occupied site. SH : active site SH group, S^- : activated active site SH group.

group is exposed to the surface without addition of Ca^{2+} ions. Conformation similar to "open form" or "permanently open form" is considered for natural μCANP, which accounts for the titration curve of SH groups in Fig. 4.

VI. ENDOGENOUS INHIBITOR AND ACTIVATOR OF CANP

In common with other protease systems, a specific proteinous CANP inhibitor (calpastatin) is found in the cytosol together with CANP. Inhibitors of chicken (42) and rabbit (43) muscle, human erythrocytes (44,45) and bovine heart (46) have been purified and their properties are summarized in Table II. Although the molecular weight and the size of subunit vary considerably, their properties are similar, i.e., the contents of aromatic amino acids are very low, and they are heatstable. CANP inhibitor forms a complex with CANP only in the presence of Ca^{2+} and inhibits the CANP activity. μ and mCANPs are inhibited at μM and mM levels of Ca^{2+}, respectively (46). This inhibition is not due to removal of Ca^{2+} or change in the sensitivity of CANP to Ca^{2+}. The inhibitor is highly specific to CANP, but various μ and mCANPs are inhibited similarly regardless of the origin: human liver inhibitor inhibits μ and mCANPs of rabbit, human, and bovine muscle

TABLE II. Properties of Purified CANP Inhibitors

	Chicken[42] muscle	Rabbit[43] muscle	Human[44,45] erythrocyte	Bovine[46] heart
Molecular weight aggregate subunit	68K	68K 34K	69–70K 250–280K	145K
Stoichiometry (inhibitor/CANP)	1	2		0.24
Heatstability	+	+	+	+
Content of aromatic amino acids	4.2%		2.2%	
Isoelectric pH			4.55	

apparently to the same extent. Various CANPs should have a common structural feature which can be recognized by the inhibitor (see Fig. 5). The stoichiometry and the reversibility of this inhibition are not yet clear. Our recent studies indicate that the inhibitor is unstable and easily degraded to small fragments by limited proteolysis during purification. The activity does not change significantly by this fragmentation. Inconsistent values for molecular weight of CANP inhibitor may be ascribed to this fragmentation.

One factor which stimulates the CANP activity has been extracted and partially purified from bovine brain (47). Although its nature is not yet understood, it increases only the maximum velocity. The complex regulatory mechanism of CANP with both inhibitor and activator indicates the importance of CANP in the cellular metabolism.

VII. BIOLOGICAL FUNCTION OF CANP

CANP has a restricted substrate specificity and lacks general proteolytic activity. This protease is therefore suitable to accomplish a specific function rather than a general function in the metabolic turnover of proteins.

Various enzymes are activated by limited proteolysis with μCANP. These include phosphorylase b kinase, phosphorylase phosphatase, glycogen synthetase, tryptophan hydroxylase and protein kinase C (for references, see 1-6). In the last case, μCANP acts only on the active form of C kinase, whereas mCANP hydrolyzes both active and inactive enzymes (48). However, the physiological meaning of this type of activation is not clear. CANP hydrolyzes several receptors or acceptor proteins (1,6). Receptors for estrogen, progesterone, glucocorticoid and epidermal growth factor are hydrolyzed to small fragments. The proteolysis changes the properties of receptors without apparent loss of binding activity, while binding capacity of glutamate receptor in rat hippocampal membrane is remarkably increased by digestion with CANP (49). Among muscle proteins, troponin, tropomyosin, myosin heavy chain and C-protein are easily hydrolyzed, while actin, myosin light chain, and M-protein are not hydrolyzed easily (1,6). Since CANP rapidly destroys the Z band which supports the myofibrillar structure and since Ca^{2+} stimulates breakdown of total proteins, it is supposed that CANP initiates turnover of intracellular proteins in vivo, especially in muscle. However, this idea needs reconsideration due to the peculiar substrate specificity and ubiquitous distribution of CANP. Many proteins related to cytoskeleton are good substrates for CANP (1,6). Tubulin, vimentin, desmin, neurofilament proteins, filamin, etc. are hydrolyzed. This may be an indication that CANP has some effects on cell shape, movement and aggregation. Although these results may be a reflection of its biological function, what must be emphasized is that most of these studies have been performed in vitro.

Why are there two CANP species? Why is mCANP which is apparently inactive in vivo present in a large amount? How does the Ca^{2+} sensitivity of mCANP change? These are important questions remaining to be answered. CANP exists mainly in cytosol, although immunofluorescent studies indicate its presence in the cell membrane (50-52). Determination and localization of μ and mCANPs and their inhibitor in tissues and cells of various physiological and pathological states will clarify the physiological role of CANP. In this respect, the recent result that μCANP is found only in the mitochondrial fraction is interesting (53).

Undoubtedly CANP plays an important role in the cellular metabolism as one of the mediators of Ca^{2+}. Thus defects in the regulatory mechanism cause abnormal increase or decrease of CANP activity and lead to various pathological states. Muscular dystrophy is probably one such example. As studies on CANP progress various diseases or pathological states which can be ascribed to its abnormal action will be found and its biological function determined.

REFERENCES

1. Murachi, T., Tanaka, K., Hatanaka, M., and Murakami, T., in "Advances in Enzyme Regulation" (G. Weber, ed.) Vol. 19, p.407. Pergamon Press, New York, 1981.
2. Ishiura, S., Life Sci. 29:1079 (1981).
3. Imahori, K., in "Calcium and Cell Function" (W. Y. Cheung, ed.) Vol. 3, p. 473. Academic Press, New York, 1982.
4. Murachi, T., Trends Biochem. Soc. 8:167 (1983).
5. Murachi, T., in "Calcium and Cell Function" (W. Y. Cheung, ed.) Vol. 4, p. 377. Academic Press, New York, 1982.
6. Kay, J., in "Proteases: Potential Role in Health and Disease" (A. Heidand, and H. Hore, eds.) in press, Plenum Press, New York.
7. Guroff, G., J. Biol. Chem. 239:149 (1964).
8. Huston, R. B., and Krebs, E. G., Biochemistry 7:2116 (1968).
9. Ishiura, S., Murofushi, H., Suzuki, K., and Imahori, K., J. Biochem. 84:225 (1978).

10. Mellgren, R. L., FEBS Lett. 109:129 (1980).
11. Suzuki, K., Ishiura, S., Tsuji, S., Katamoto, T., Sugita, H., and Imahori, K., FEBS Lett. 104:355 (1979).
12. Azanza, J. L., Raymond, J., Robin, J. M., Cottin, P., and Ducastang, A., Biochem. J. 183:339 (1979).
13. Tsuji, S., and Imahori, K., J. Biochem. 90:233 (1981).
14. Mellgren, R. L., Repetti, A., Muck, T. C., and Easly, J., J. Biol. Chem. 257:7203 (1982).
15. Dayton, W. R., Goll, D. E., Zeece, M. G., Robson, R. M., and Reville, W. J., Biochemistry 15:2150 (1976).
16. Corall, D. E., and DeMartino, G. N., J. Biol. Chem. 258:5660 (1983).
17. Otsuka, Y., and Tanaka, H., Biochem. Biophys. Res. Commun. 111:700 (1983).
18. Tolnai, S., Can. J. Biochem. 59:242 (1981).
19. Hara, K., Ichihara, Y., and Takahashi, K., J. Biochem. 93:1435 (1983).
20. Hathaway, D. R., Werth, D. K., and Haeberle, J. R., J. Biol. Chem. 257:9072 (1982).
21. Yoshimura, N., Kikuchi, T., Sasaki, T., Kitahara, A., Hatanaka, M., and Murachi, T., J. Biol. Chem. 258:8883 (1983).
22. Malik, M. N., Fenko, M. D., Iqubal, K., and Wisniewski, H. M., J. Biol. Chem. 258:8955 (1983).
23. Truglia, J. A., and Stracher, A., Biochem. Biophys. Res. Commun. 100:814 (1981).
24. Yoshida, N., Weksler, B., and Nachman, R., J. Biol. Chem. 258:7168 (1983).
25. Kubota, S., and Suzuki, K., Biomed. Res. 3:699 (1982).
26. Inomata, M., Hayashi, M., Nakamura, M., Imahori, K., and Kawashima, S., J. Biochem. 93:291 (1983).
27. Dayton, W. R., Schollmeyer, J. V., Lepley, R. A., and Cortes, L. R., Biochim. Biophys. Acta 659:48 (1981).
28. Melloni, E., Sparatore, B., Salamino, F., Michetti, M., and Pontremoli, S., Biochem. Biophys. Res. Commun. 106:731 (1982).
29. Tsujinaka, T., Shiba, E., Kambayashi, J., and Kosaki, G., Biochem. Intern. 6:71 (1983).
30. Nelson, W. J., and Traub, P., J. Biol. Chem. 257:5544 (1982).
31. Ishiura, S., Sugita, H., Suzuki, K., and Imahori, K., J. Biochem. 86:579 (1979).
32. Murachi, T., Hatanaka, M., Yamamoto, Y., Nakamura, N., and Tanaka, K., Biochem. Intern. 2:651 (1981).
33. Wheelock, M. J., J. Biol. Chem. 257:12471 (1982).
34. Dayton, W. R., Biochim. Biophys. Acta 709:166 (1982).
35. Suzuki, K., Tsuji, S., and Ishiura, S., FEBS Lett. 136:119 (1981).
36. Suzuki, K., J. Biochem. 93:1305 (1983).

37. Suzuki, K., Hayashi, H., Hayashi, T., and Iwai, K., FEBS Lett. 152:67 (1983).

38. Suzuki, K., Tsuji, S., Kubota, S., Kimura, Y., and Imahori, K., J. Biochem. 90:275 (1981).

39. Suzuki, K., Tsuji, S., Ishiura, S., Kimura, Y., Kubota, S., and Imahori, K., J. Biochem. 90:1787 (1983).

40. Suzuki, K., and Tsuji, S., FEBS Lett. 140:16 (1983).

41. Suzuki, K., and Ishiura, S., J. Biochem. 93:1463 (1983).

42. Ishiura, S., Tsuji, S., Murofushi, H., and Suzuki, K., Biochim. Biophys. Acta 701:216 (1982).

43. Takahashi-Nakamura, M., Tsuji, S., Suzuki, K., and Imahori, K., J. Biochem. 90:1583 (1981).

44. Takano, E., and Murachi, T., J. Biochem. 92:2021 (1982).

45. Melloni, B., Sparatore, B., Salamino, F., Michetti, M., and Pontremoli, S., Biochem. Biophys. Res. Commun. 107:1053 (1982).

46. Mellgren, R. L., and Carr, T. C., Arch. Biochem. Biophys. 225:779 (1983).

47. Demartino, G. N., and Blumenthal, D. K., Biochemistry 21:4297 (1982).

48. Kishimoto, A., Kajikawa, N., Shiota, M., and Nishizuka, Y., J. Biol. Chem. 258:1156 (1983).

49. Vargas, F. and Costa, E., in "Advances in Biochemical Psychopharmacology" (G. DiChiara, and G. L. Gessa, eds.) Vol. 27, p. 307. Raven Press, New York, 1981.

50. Ishiura, S., Sugita, H., Nonaka, I., and Imahori, K., J. Biochem. 87:343 (1980).

51. Dayton, W. R., and Schollmeyer, J. V., Exptl. Cell Res. 136:423 (1981).

52. Barth, R., and Elce, J. S., Am. J. Physiol. 240:E493 (1981).

53. Beer, D. G., Hjelle, J. J., Petersen, D. R., and Malkinson, A. M., Biochem. Biophys. Res. Commun. 109:1276 (1982).

CALCIUM IONS AND THE REGULATION OF INTRACELLULAR PROTEIN BREAKDOWN IN MUSCLE

Vickie E. Baracos
Robert E. Greenberg[1]
Alfred L. Goldberg

Department of Physiology and Biophysics
Harvard Medical School
Boston, Mass.

I. INTRODUCTION

In skeletal muscle, rates of protein degradation, like rates of protein synthesis, are precisely regulated, and a number of physiological and pathological factors has been shown to alter overall rates of protein breakdown in this tissue, including insulin, thyroid hormones, glucocorticoids, and muscular activity (1-5). Furthermore, the overall rate of proteolysis can be an important determinant of muscle size (1,3,4). For example, during fever or after denervation, there can be a marked acceleration of muscle protein breakdown which results in muscle atrophy (6-8). Because skeletal muscle constitutes the major protein reservoir in mammals, protein degradation in muscle also is crucial in the mobilization of amino acids for energy production during fasting (9).

Recent advances in our knowledge about the regulation of protein breakdown has been made largely through the study of isolated muscles incubated _in vitro_ and perfused hindlimbs (2,3,6,7,10). Simple techniques have been introduced for monitoring overall rates of protein synthesis and breakdown in these isolated tissues (10). When rat muscles are incubated _in vitro_, their rates of protein degradation exceed rates of

---

[1]Present address: Department of Pediatrics, University of New Mexico, School of Medicine, Albuquerque, New Mexico

CALCIUM REGULATION
IN BIOLOGICAL SYSTEMS

227

synthesis.   This net proteolysis falls upon addition of
various factors found in vivo, but absent in Krebs–Ringer buffer: insulin, glucose, and leucine (but no other amino
acid)(11).   In addition, if the muscles are maintained under
passive   tension   (5,12),   they   approach   nitrogen   balance.
Although appreciable progress has been made in defining how
insulin, nutrients, and contractile activity can affect muscle
protein breakdown, the intracellular mechanisms responsible
for these alterations in degradative rates remain unclear.   In
fact, our knowledge about the biochemical pathways and the
intracellular sites of protein degradation is still quite
limited in all mammalian cells, especially skeletal muscle.
     Research in our laboratory is attempting to clarify the
physiological factors regulating protein turnover in muscle
and to elucidate the intracellular mechanisms responsible for
the breakdown of cell proteins.   It is well established that
Ca^{2+} ions play a central role in the regulation of a variety
of cellular processes ranging from muscle contraction to the
secretion of intracellular vesicles (19–21).   Recently, evidence has accumulated from our work (13–15) and from other
laboratories (16–18) that Ca^{2+} can also play a critical role
in the control of protein breakdown in skeletal muscle.
Involvement of Ca^{2+} in the control of protein breakdown is not
only of scientific interest but is also of potential medical
import, since in certain pathological conditions where muscular atrophy is pronounced (e.g. muscular dystrophy, denervation, burns), muscle cells have been reported to contain
high levels of Ca^{2+} (8,22–24).   Since this ion triggers
contractile activity in muscle (20), it may also play a role
in the coupling of mechanical activity to the control of
muscle size (e.g. in work–induced hypertrophy or disuse
atrophy).

II. EFFECTS OF Ca^{2+} ON MUSCLE PROTEIN TURNOVER

     Recently, we have attempted to define more precisely the
influence of Ca^{2+} and other ions on protein turnover in skeletal muscle and to investigate the possible mechanisms by which
Ca^{2+} influences this process (13–15).   Kameyama and Etlinger
(16) first demonstrated that when entry of Ca^{2+} into muscle
was   increased   by   the   addition   of   the   ionophore, A_{23187},
overall protein degradation increased.   This phenomenon has
been studied further in several laboratories (13,17,18) and
shown (13) to occur independently of any change in protein
synthesis (Table I).   Because of the multiple actions of the
ionophore (25), it was initially unclear if the accelerated
protein breakdown was indicative of a physiological role for

Table I. Effects of Ca^{2+} and Ca^{2+} Plus A_{23187}
on Protein Turnover in Rat Diaphragm

Treatment	Protein Synthesis	Protein Degradation (nmol tyr/mg/2 hr)	Net Protein Degradation
Expt. I			
Ca^{2+}	0.184 ± 0.029	0.627 ± 0.050	-0.433 ± 0.039
$Ca^{2+} + A_{23187}$	0.252 ± 0.026	0.967 ± 0.056	-0.709 ± 0.039
Change	NS	+53%*	+64%*
Expt. II			
None	0.069 ± 0.003	0.250 ± 0.009	-0.181 ± 0.001
Ca^{2+}	0.072 ± 0.004	0.642 ± 0.028	-0.570 ± 0.027
Change	NS	+157%**	+215%**

*$p < 0.01$; **$p < 0.001$; NS = not significant (n=7).
Quarter diaphragms were preincubated 30 min. in KRB containing the stated additions. Ca^{2+} was added at a final concentration of 2.58 mM. Muscles were transferred to fresh media of the same composition and incubated for 2 hr. Rates of protein synthesis, protein degradation, and net protein degradation were measured as described by Tischler et al. (26).

Ca^{2+} in regulating protein turnover or a pathological response of the tissue to the ionophore. However, even in the absence of the ionophore, the level of Ca^{2+} in the incubation medium also influences rates of protein breakdown (14, Table I). Normally, isolated muscles are maintained in Krebs-Ringer bicarbonate buffer (KRB) (11), which contains 2.58 mM Ca^{2+}, and under these conditions, the tissues are highly catabolic. However, when rat muscles are incubated in Ca^{2+}-free buffer, the overall rate of protein breakdown was 60% lower in diaphragm (Table I, Fig. 1) and 35% lower in extensor digitorum longus (Table II) and soleus than when they were in normal Krebs-Ringer bicarbonate buffer (14). To prepare the Ca^{2+}-free media, this ion was simply omitted from the KRB or the HEPES buffers. In our studies, EGTA was not utilized to lower intracellular Ca^{2+} concentrations further, since this agent can reduce ATP and phosphocreatine content of muscles and cause leakage of cell enzymes (17).
In order to study systematically the effects of extra-

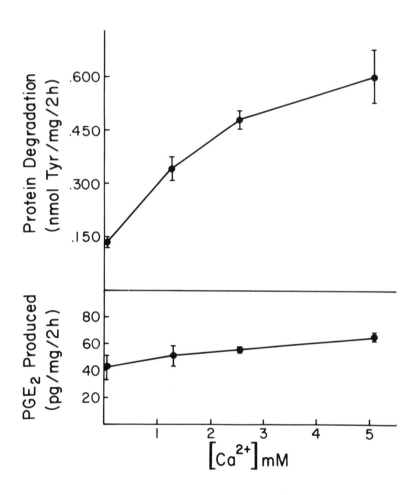

FIGURE 1.   Effect of extracellular Ca^{2+} on protein degradation and prostaglandin production by diaphragm muscle.   Rat
quarter diaphragms were incubated in HEPES buffer in the presence of cycloheximide.   Muscles were preincubated for 30 min
at the stated Ca^{2+} concentrations, then transferred to fresh
media of the same composition and incubated for a further 2
hr.   The production of PGE_2 by the muscles was estimated by
radioimmunoassay of the PGE_2 released into the incubation
medium, as previously described (6,13,50).   (n=7).

Table II. Influence of Ca2+ on Protein Degradation, ATP and
Phosphocreatine in Rat Extensor Digitorum Longus
Muscle

	$[Ca^{2+}]$ (mM)			
	0	1.29	2.58	5.16

Expt. I

Protein
Degrada-
tion   0.156±0.003 0.195±0.005* 0.238±0.009* 0.262±0.006*
(nmol
tyr/mg/2 hr)

Expt. II

ATP
(μmol/gm) 3.42 ± 0.23 3.83 ± 0.29 3.61 ± 0.17 3.20 ± 0.18

Phospho-
creatine   7.06 ± 0.78 6.84 ± 0.49 6.76 ± 0.43 6.60 ± 0.74
(μmol/gm)

*Difference from 0 mM Ca^{2+}, $p < 0.001$ (n=7).

Muscles were preincubated for 30 min in HEPES buffer con
taining 0.5 mM cycloheximide at the stated Ca^{2+} concentrations, then transferred to fresh media and incubated for
further 2 hr. ATP and phosphocreatine contents were determined according to the method described by Lowry (51). No
significant differences were observed in ATP or phosphocreatine content.

cellular Ca^{2+} on muscle protein turnover, rat muscles were
incubated in buffers containing different concentrations of
$CaCl_2$, and protein degradation was estimated by determining
the rate of appearance of tyrosine in the medium, which
reflects the rate of production of tyrosine from cell proteins
(11,26). As shown in Fig. 1, proteolysis in the rat diaphragm
was lowest when Ca^{2+} was omitted from the medium. This process increased up to 3 to 4 fold as the Ca^{2+} concentration was
raised to 5.16 mM. It is noteworthy that protein breakdown is
very sensitive to changes in Ca^{2+} levels between 1 and 2 mM,
the concentration range found in vivo. At the concentration
of Ca^{2+} usually used in vitro (2.58 mM), proteolysis was

3-fold greater than in Ca^{2+}-free medium and also greater than at the Ca^{2+} concentrations found in extracellular fluids. Thus the negative protein balance exhibited by such isolated muscles <u>in vitro</u> may in part result from this enhancement of proteolysis by Ca^{2+}.

This ion stimulated protein breakdown similarly in the soleus, an oxidative-slow muscle, and the extensor digitorum longus, a glycolytic-fast muscle, although in both, the response to Ca^{2+} was less than in the diaphragm (14) for reasons that are not clear. One useful criterion of tissue viability is the intracellular content of ATP and phosphocreatine, neither of which was affected by the removal of Ca^{2+} from the medium or by Ca^{2+} concentration up to 5.16 mM (Table II). Therefore, the associated changes in protein degradation do not appear to be a nonspecific or toxic effect. Furthermore, over this wide range of Ca^{2+} concentrations, protein synthetic rates did not vary (14). Therefore, with increasing Ca^{2+} concentrations, the tissues showed a marked negative nitrogen balance as a consequence of the more rapid proteolysis.

III. INVOLVEMENT OF LYSOSOMAL PROTEASES IN THIS RESPONSE

It is now well established that mammalian cells contain multiple pathways for protein breakdown (1,2,27,28), which can serve distinct physiological functions. The lysosome is an important site for protein breakdown in mammalian cells, although its contribution to overall proteolysis seems to vary with the physiological conditions (1). This organelle contains a high concentration of proteolytic enzymes, such as cathepsins A, B, C, D, H and L (1). At present the mechanisms by which cytoplasmic proteins enter and are degraded in lysosomes are not clear. A variety of studies in liver and fibroblasts suggest that this process involves the engulfment of areas of cytoplasm in membraneous vesicles, which then fuse with lysosomes to form "autophagic vacuoles" (27,29,30). Particularly useful tools to clarify the physiological role of lysosomes in muscle and other tissues are the protease inhibitors of microbial origin: the peptide aldehydes (e.g. leupeptin) (31) isolated from Actinomyces by Umezawa and colleagues and the epoxide derivatives of E-64 (especially Ep-475) (32) introduced by Hanada and coworkers.

To test if lysosomes are involved in the stimulation of protein degradation by Ca^{2+}, we employed Ep-475 (E-64-C) and leupeptin to inhibit lysosomal thiol proteases. These agents are irreversible inhibitors of cathepsins B, H and L (31,32). We have previously found that these compounds can enter intact muscles, inactivate lysosomal enzymes, and decrease overall protein breakdown (13,33,34). In fact, they have been utilized to implicate lysosomes in various physiological responses. These agents have proven particularly effective against the acceleration of proteolysis in muscle induced with prostaglandin E_2 (13) or by interleukin-1 (leukocytic pyrogen) (6,15). Therefore, these responses appear to involve an activation of the lysosomal pathway. Upon incubation with these inhibitors, cathepsin B activity within the muscle decreased by greater than 80% (13,14). As shown in Table III, the increase in protein breakdown induced by the addition of Ca^{2+} to the medium or by Ca^{2+} ionophores (13) was also markedly inhibited by Ep-475 or leupeptin (14). By contrast, in Ca^{2+}-free media, inactivation of cathepsin B did not cause any reduction in protein breakdown. These findings suggest that the protein breakdown in the absence of Ca^{2+} occurs by a nonlysosomal process, which remains to be identified.

Table III. The Effect of Ep-475 and Leupeptin on the Stimulation of Protein Breakdown by Ca^{2+}

Treatment	Protein Degradation (nmol tyr/mg/2 hr)		
	$-Ca^{2+}$	$+Ca^{2+}$	
None	0.164 ± 0.017	0.327 ± 0.047	+99%[**]
Ep-475	0.171 ± 0.013	0.214 ± 0.025	NS
Difference	NS	-35%[*]	
None	0.226 ± 0.009	0.532 ± 0.013	+135%[**]
Leupeptin	0.248 ± 0.006	0.245 ± 0.007	NS
Difference	NS	-54%[**]	

[*]$p < 0.025$; [**]$p < 0.001$ (n=7); NS = Not significant.

Quarter diaphragms were incubated in HEPES buffer in the presence of cycloheximide. The preincubation and incubation periods were 90 min. Muscles were preincubared in the presence or absence of Ep-475 (25 μM) or leupeptin (30 μM). To facilitate inhibitor entry, Ca^{2+} (1.29 mM) was also present in the preincubation medium. During the subsequent incubation, muscles were incubated with or without Ep-475 or leupeptin in the presence of either 0 or 5.16 mM Ca^{2+}. In the muscles treated with Ep-475 or leupeptin, cathepsin B activity was inhibited more than 80%.

Most likely Ca^{2+} activates some step essential in the lysosome's proteolytic function (e.g. acidification), in the formation of autophagic vacuoles, or in the fusion of lyso- somes with autophagic vacuoles. In accord with the latter view, Altstiel and Branton have shown that Ca^{2+} is essential for the fusion of coated vesicles with lysosomes (35). Also we did find that some extracellular Ca^{2+} is essential for Ep-475 to gain access to the lysosomal protease (14). This finding, which complicated our experimental design (Table III, legend), may indicate that Ca^{2+} is essential for uptake of materials into lysosomes from either the cytosol or from endocytosed vacuoles. Since these studies on muscle were completed, Grinde, using very different approaches, has pre- sented evidence that Ca^{2+} ions also play an important role in intralysosomal proteolysis in rat hepatocytes (36). In addi- tion, our own studies (14) indicate that Ca^{2+} may also stimulate proteolysis in muscle by a nonlysosomal mechanism.

An alternative possibility is that Ca^{2+} affects the Ca^{2+}-activated protease (calpain) (37), as discussed in detail in the prior report. The cytoplasm of skeletal muscle con- tains a Ca^{2+}-activated protease (37), whose interesting enzy- mological properties have been carefully studied, but whose physiological function remains unclear. Prior reports suggested that the Ca^{2+} ionophores may enhance proteolysis in muscle by activating this enzyme (16,17). We have found that in the incubated muscles the sulfhydryl reagent, mersalyl, could completely inactivate the Ca^{2+}-dependent protease without affecting the tissue's lysosomal thiol proteases, even though mersalyl can inactivate both enzymes in tissue homoge- nates (13). Treatment with this agent does not reduce overall rates of protein breakdown in the muscle or, more importantly, the stimulation of proteolysis by extracellular Ca^{2+} or Ca^{2+} ionophores (Tables IV, V). These findings indicate that the Ca^{2+}-activated protease is not essential for overall protein breakdown in the muscle or for the enhancement of this process by Ca^{2+}, both of which require cathepsin B and perhaps other lysosomal proteases.

IV. SPECIFICITY FOR Ca^{2+}

Many of the physiological effects of Ca^{2+}, such as the release of secretory vesicles from nerves and glands, can be mimicked by Sr^{2+} and Ba^{2+} and inhibited by Mg^{2+} (19,38,39). When Sr^{2+}, Ba^{2+} or Mn^{2+} were added to media lacking divalent cations, protein degradation increased, although the ability of these ions to enhance proteolysis was less than that pro-

Table IV. Effect of Mersalyl on the Stimulation of Protein Breakdown by Ca^{2+}

Addition	Protein Degradation (nmol tyr/mg/2 hr)		
	$-Ca^{2+}$	$+Ca^{2+}$	% Increase
None	0.265 ± 0.022	0.615 ± 0.018	+132[*]
Mersalyl	0.324 ± 0.017	0.776 ± 0.035	+140[*]

[*]$p < 0.001$ (n=7).

Quarter diaphragms were incubated in HEPES buffer in the presence of cycloheximide. Muscles were preincubated 1.0 hr, then transferred to fresh media and incubated for a further 2 hr. Mersalyl (0.2 mM) and Ca^{2+} (5.16 mM) were added to both preincubation and incubation media, as indicated. In the muscles treated with mersalyl, the activity of the Ca^{2+}-activated protease was almost completely inhibited.

Table V. Factors Affecting the Enhancement of Protein Breakdown in Skeletal Muscle by Ca^{2+}

1.	Ep-475	Inhibits
2.	Leupeptin	Inhibits
3.	Indomethacin	No Effect
4.	Mersalyl (Inactivates Ca^{2+}-activated protease)	No Effect
5.	W 7 (Calmodulin antagonist)	No Effect
6.	Ca^{2+}-channel blockers (Verapamil, Nifedipine)	No Effect
7.	Microtubule/microfilament antagonists (Colchicine, Vinblastine, Cytochalasin B)	No Effect
8.	Metalloendoprotease inhibitors (Phosphoramidon, 1,10-Phenanthroline)	No Effect

duced by Ca^{2+} at equimolar concentrations (Table VI). At concentrations found in plasma (1-2 mM), Mg^{2+} failed to increase protein breakdown, although it did have a small effect at much higher concentrations. When Ca^{2+} was also present in the media, the addition of Mg^{2+} at physiological concentrations (1-2 mM) or higher inhibited the increase in protein breakdown induced by Ca^{2+} or by the Ca^{2+} ionophore, A_{23187}. Thus, in vivo, extracellular Mg^{2+} may retard protein breakdown in muscle by inhibiting the stimulatory effects of Ca^{2+} on proteolysis. It is interesting that in isolated hepatocytes (36), unlike in muscle, Mg^{2+} seems to act like Ca^{2+} in promoting proteolysis, and the two ions have additive rather than opposing effects. The basis for these tissue differences will be an interesting topic for future study.

Table VI. Effect of Divalent Cations on Protein Degradation in Rat Diaphragm

	Divalent Cation	Protein Degradation (nmol tyr/mg/2 hr)	Increase
Expt. I	None	0.275 ± 0.015	
	Ca^{2+} (2.5 mM)	0.626 ± 0.043	+128%**
	Mg^{2+} (2.5 mM)	0.289 ± 0.010	NS
	Mn^{2+} (2.5 mM)	0.338 ± 0.012	+23%*
Expt. II	None	0.202 ± 0.009	
	Ca^{2+} (2.5 mM)	0.443 ± 0.030	+119%**
	Sr^{2+} (2.5 mM)	0.304 ± 0.022	+50%**
	Ba^{2+} (2.5 mM)	0.308 ± 0.023	+52%**
Expt. III	None	0.229 ± 0.001	
	Mg^{2+} (6.25 mM)	0.231 ± 0.020	NS
	Mg^{2+} (12.5 mM)	0.316 ± 0.020	+38%*
	Mn^{2+} (12.5 mM)	0.514 ± 0.033	+124%**

*$p < 0.05$; **$p < 0.001$ (n=7); NS = Not significant.
Quarter diaphragms were incubated in Ca^{2+}- and Mg^{2+}-free HEPES buffer in the presence of cycloheximide. Divalent cations were added to both preincubation and incubation media, as indicated.

V. POSSIBLE MECHANISMS OF Ca^{2+}-INDUCED PROTEOLYSIS

At present, the mechanisms whereby Ca^{2+} in the medium promotes intracellular proteolysis are uncertain. Our studies have not determined definitively whether Ca^{2+} must enter the cell to influence intracellular proteolysis or whether it may do so by acting on the cell membrane. An intracellular site of action seems most likely, in light of the similar effects induced by extracellular Ca^{2+} and the ionophores (13,14). It would be very interesting to know how extracellular Ca^{2+} influences the free cytosolic Ca^{2+} concentration. Studies with Ca^{2+}-specific microelectrodes have indicated that in frog muscle, cytosolic Ca^{2+} falls 3-fold when the tissue is suspended in Ca^{2+}-free buffers (40). The availability of similar data on these isolated rat skeletal muscle preparations would be particularly informative for understanding the mechanisms of the Ca^{2+} effect on proteolysis.

To explore how Ca^{2+} may stimulate proteolysis, we have investigated several possible mediators of this response (Table V):

1) One group of molecules that may influence protein degradation in muscle and may mediate hormonal effects is the prostaglandins (PG) and in particular PGE_2. Rodemann and Goldberg (33) showed that PGE_2 can accelerate proteolysis in skeletal and cardiac muscle. We have recently obtained evidence that PGE_2 may be important in accelerating proteolysis in disease states. For example, in sepsis and fever, protein breakdown in muscle seems to be stimulated by the circulating polypeptide released by mononuclear phagocytes, interleukin-1 (leukocytic pyrogen) (6,41, see below). The resulting acceleration of proteolysis is mediated by PGE_2 (6). Similarly, Ca^{2+} or the Ca^{2+} ionophore possibly could enhance proteolysis by enhancing PGE_2 production. Our previous work (13) had shown that the Ca^{2+} ionophore, A_{23187}, causes a marked stimulation of PGE_2 synthesis in these muscles, and experiments with indomethacin had suggested the rise in PGE_2 was important in the enhancement of proteolysis. Simply increasing the external Ca^{2+} concentrations in the medium also causes muscle production of PGE_2 to rise significantly (Fig. 1). However, this effect seems to be independent of and not necessary for the enhancement of proteolysis, since Ca^{2+} was found to stimulate proteolysis equally effectively when PGE_2 synthesis was prevented by indomethacin, an inhibitor of arachidonic acid cyclooxygenase (Table V). Because of the disagreement with the prior findings (13), we carefully reexamined the suggested involvement of PGE_2 in the response to A_{23187}. In an extensive series of experiments indomethacin did not reduce the ionophore's ability to stimulate proteolysis, in contrast to

what had been observed consistently before. Although PGE_2 may be an important regulator of proteolysis under certain conditions (6), these observations clearly show that Ca^{2+} and the Ca^{2+} ionophore can promote proteolysis independently of changes in prostaglandin formation.

2) Many of the physiological effects of Ca^{2+} within cells involve the binding of this ion to calmodulin (42), which regulates the function of a large variety of cell enzymes, as discussed extensively in this book. To determine whether calmodulin is also playing an important role in the regulation of proteolysis, we have used the calmodulin antagonist, W7 (43,44). However, neither this agent nor its inactive analog, W5, affected the stimulation of proteolysis by Ca^{2+} ions (14, Table V).

3) To determine whether Ca^{2+} entry into the muscle cells via voltage-dependent Ca^{2+} channels results in increased protein breakdown, we studied the effects of nifedipine or verapamil (45). Neither of these Ca^{2+} channel blockers affected proteolysis in the presence of Ca^{2+} (14, Table V).

4) Microfilaments and microtubules have been suggested to play an essential role in several Ca^{2+}-dependent cellular processes (19,21,29) including autophagic vacuole formation (46,47). Although it has been reported that microtubular inhibitors can block increased proteolysis under certain conditions (46), we failed to find any significant inhibition of Ca^{2+}-stimulated proteolysis in the muscle cells with colchicine, vinblastine, or cytochalasin B (14, Table V).

5) It has recently been reported that two Ca^{2+}-dependent processes, the fusion of myoblasts into myotubes (48) and the release of transmitters from the neuromuscular junction (49), require the activity of a metalloendoprotease sensitive to 1,10-phenanthroline and phosphoramidon. We therefore used these inhibitors at concentrations that affect these other Ca^{2+}-dependent processes, but these agents did not affect the activation of proteolysis by Ca^{2+} (14, Table V).

VI. CONCLUSIONS

These experiments (14) have demonstrated an important regulatory function of Ca^{2+} and Mg^{2+} ions on protein breakdown. Our studies thus far have clearly implicated the lysosomal pathway in the response to Ca^{2+} but have not provided any clear insights concerning this ion's mechanism of action. It is hoped that further information on the mode of regulation of lysosomal protein breakdown by Ca^{2+} will help us clarify the rate-limiting steps in this process.

The importance of these effects of Ca^{2+} under different

physiological and pathological conditions should be an
interesting and fruitful area for future study. For example,
we have shown that the activation of muscle protein breakdown
in fever or sepsis may be signaled by leukocytic pyrogen,
which appears identical to interleukin-1 (6,41). This polypeptide, which is released by mononuclear phagocytes, not only
acts on the hypothalamus to induce fever but can also act
directly on muscle to promote PGE_2 Production and intralysosomal protein breakdown (6, Fig. 2). This acceleration of
proteolysis is markedly reduced in Ca^{2+}-free medium (14).
Similarly, when muscles are removed from febrile animals and
incubated in vitro, they show up to 2-fold more rapid protein
breakdown than controls, and this response also depends on the

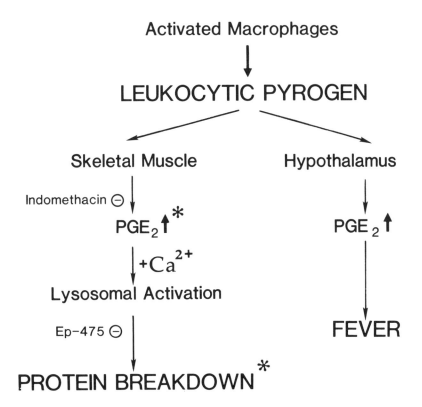

FIGURE 2. Proposed mechanism for the effects of leukocytic pyrogen (interleukin-1) in inducing fever and muscle protein breakdown. *Augmented response at febrile temperatures.

presence of Ca^{2+} in the medium (Fagan, J. and Goldberg, A. L., manuscript in preparation).

It is intriguing to suggest that alterations in Ca^{2+} entry into the muscle or the redistribution of Ca^{2+} ions stored within the sarcoplasmic reticulum may be responsible for the activation of protein breakdown in these muscles and in other physiological conditions. In fact, in recent studies, we have found that inhibitors of Ca^{2+} release from the endoplasmic reticulum can reduce protein breakdown under these conditions (Baracos, V. E. and Goldberg, A. L., unpublished observations). The physiological importance of such findings and their biochemical basis remain to be elucidated.

REFERENCES

1. Wildenthal, K. (ed.), in "Degradative Processes in Skeletal and Cardiac Muscle", Elsevier/North Holland, Amsterdam, 1980.
2. Waterlow, J. C., Garlick, P. J., and Millward, D. J., "Protein Turnover in Mammalian Tissues and the Whole Body", Elsevier/North Holland, Amsterdam, 1978.
3. Goldberg, A. L., Tischler, M. E., DeMartino, G., and Griffin, G., Fed. Proc. 39:31 (1980).
4. Tischler, M. E., Life Sci. 28:2569 (1981).
5. Goldberg, A. L., Etlinger, J. D., Goldspink, D. F., and Jablecki, C., Med. and Sci. in Sports 7:1248 (1975).
6. Baracos, V. E., Rodemann, H. P., Dinarello, C. A., and Goldberg, A. L., New Eng. J. Med. 308:553 (1983).
7. Clowes, G. H. A., George, B. C., Villee, C. A., Jr., and Saravis, C. A., New Eng. J. Med. 308:545 (1983).
8. Goldspink, D. F., Biochem. J. 156:71 (1976).
9. Ruderman, N. B., Ann. Rev. Med. 26:245 (1975).
10. Goldberg, A. L., Martel, S. M., and Kushmerick, M. J., Methods Enzymol. 39:82 (1975).
11. Fulks, R., Li, J. B., and Goldberg, A. L., J. Biol. Chem. 250:290 (1975).
12. Etlinger, J. D., Kameyama, T., Toner, K., Van der Westhuyzen, D., and Matsumoto, K., in "Plasticity of Muscle" (D. Pette, ed.), p. 541. Walter de Gruyter, New York, 1980.
13. Rodemann, H. P., Waxman, L., and Goldberg, A. L., J. Biol. Chem. 257:8716 (1982).
14. Greenberg, R. E., Baracos, V. E., Freedman, N., and Goldberg, A. L., submitted for publication (1984).
15. Goldberg, A. L., Baracos, V. E., Rodemann, P., Waxman, L., and Dinarello, C. A., Fed. Proc. 43:1301 (1984).

16. Kameyama, T., and Etlinger, J. D., Nature 279:344 (1979).
17. Sugden, P. H., Biochem. J. 190:593 (1980).
18. Lewis, S. E. M., Anderson, P., and Goldspink, D. F., Biochem. J. 204:257 (1982).
19. Rubin, R. P., "Calcium and Cellular Secretion", Plenum Press, New York, 1982.
20. Peachey, L., Adrian, R., and Geiger, S. R., "Handbook of Physiology: Skeletal Muscle", American Physiological Soc., Bethesda, 1983.
21. Cheung, W. Y., "Calcium and Cell Function", Academic Press, New York, 1983.
22. Engel, A. G., Mokri, B., Jerusalem, F., Sakakibara, H., and Paulson, O. B., in "Pathogenesis of Human Muscular Dystrophies" (L. P. Rowland, ed.), p. 310. Excerpta Medica, Amsterdam, 1977.
23. Joffe, M., Savage, N., and Isaacs, H., Biochem. J. 196:663 (1981).
24. Rourke, A. W., J. Cell Physiol. 86:343 (1975).
25. Reed, P. W., and Lardy, H. A., J. Biol. Chem. 247:6970 (1972).
26. Tischler, M. E., Desautels, M., and Goldberg, A. L., J. Biol. Chem. 257:1613 (1982).
27. Hershko, A., and Ciechanover, A., Ann. Rev. Biochem. 51:335 (1982).
28. Goldberg, A. L., and St. John, A. C., Ann. Rev., Biochem. 45:747 (1976).
29. Kominami, E., Hashida, S., Khairallah, E. A., and Katunuma, N., J. Biol. Chem. 258:6093 (1983).
30. Mortimore, G. E., Nutri. Rev. 40:1 (1982).
31. Umezawa, H., Methods Enzymol. 45:678 (1976).
32. Hanada, K., Tamai, M., Yamagishi, M., Ohmura, S., Sawada, J., and Tanaka, I., Agric. Biol. Chem. 42:523 (1978).
33. Rodemann, H. P., and Goldberg, A. L., J. Biol. Chem. 257:1632 (1982).
34. Libby, P., and Goldberg, A. L., J. Cell Physiol. 107:185 (1981).
35. Altstiel, L., and Branton, D., Cell 32:921 (1983).
36. Grinde, B., Biochem. J. 216:529 (1983).
37. Waxman, L., Methods Enzymol. 80:664 (1982).
38. Fatt, P., and Ginsborg, B. L., J. Physiol. (London) 142:516 (1958).
39. Nakayato, Y., and Onoda, Y., J. Physiol. (London) 305:59 (1980).
40. Lopez, J. R., Alamo, L., Caputo, C., Dipolo, R., and Vergara, J., Biophys. J. 43:1 (1983).
41. Dinarello, C. A., Rev. Infec. Dis. 6:5 (1984).
42. Cheung, W. Y., Science 207:19 (1980).
43. Nelson, G. A., Andrews, J. L., and Karnovsky, M. J., J. Cell Biol. 95:771 (1982).

44. Hidaka, H., Sasaki, K., Tanaka, T., Endo, T., Ohno, S., Fujii, Y., and Nagata, T., Proc. Natl. Acad. Sci. USA 78:4354 (erratum 7844) (1981).

45. Triggle, D. J., in "New Perspectives on Calcium Antagonists" (B. B. Weiss, ed.), p. 1. Waverly Press, Baltimore, 1981.

46. Amenta, J. S., and Brocher, S. C., Life Sci. 28:1195 (1981).

47. Kovacs, A. T., Reith, A., and Seglen, P. O., Exp. Cell Res. 137:191 (1982).

48. Couch, C. B., Strittmatter, W. J., Cell 32:257 (1983).

49. Baxter, D. A., Johnston, D., Strittmatter, W. J., Proc. Natl. Acad. Sci. USA 80:4174 (1983).

50. Jaffe, B. M., and Behrman, H. R., "Methods of Hormone Radioimmunoassay", p. 19. Academic Press, New York, 1974.

51. Lowry, O. H., and Passonneau, J. V., "A Flexible System of Enzymatic Analysis", Academic Press, New York, 1972.

Ca-ACTIVATED NEUTRAL PROTEASE
IN PHYSIOLOGICAL AND PATHOLOGICAL CONDITIONS[1]

Hideo Sugita
Shoichi Ishiura
Keiko Kamakura
Hirofumi Nakase
Koichi Hagiwara
Ikuya Nonaka*

Division of Neuromuscular Research
and
*Division of Ultrastructural Research
National Center for Nervous, Mental
and Muscular Disorders
Kodaira, Tokyo

Ken-ichi Tomomatsu

First Department of Internal Medicine
Faculty of Medicine
University of Tokyo
Tokyo

I. INTRODUCTION

Many investigators now agree that in most tissues, proteolysis probably involves both lysosomal and non-lysosomal
processes. There remains, however, much debate on their rela-

---

[1]This work was supported in part by Grant No. 82-04 from
the National Center for Nervous, Mental and Muscular Disorders
(NCNMMD), a Grant-in-Aid of New Drug Development from the
Ministry of Health and Welfare and grants from the Ministry of
Education, Science and Culture, Japan.

tive importance. Since Ca-activated neutral protease (CANP)
was purified from skeletal muscle, similar enzymes have been
isolated from virtually every cell type, such as brain, liver,
kidney, smooth and cardiac muscles, blood cells including
erythrocytes and platelets and oviduct.

The cells have two types of CANP, m-CANP and μ-CANP
following Suzuki's nomenclature (1), and their ratio differs
in different cells. Human red cell has predominantly μ-CANP
(2). The cells also have endogenous inhibitors. Interestingly enough, liver contains more inhibitor than CANP, while the
reverse is true in brain according to Murachi and his group
(3). Therefore, the function of CANP must involve a very complicated regulation mechanism under both physiological and
pathological conditions.

II. LOCALIZATION OF CANP IN THE CELL

Several conflicting data have been reported as a result of
immunofluorescent localization studies of this enzyme in the
muscle. Barth and Elce (4) reported that the enzyme was
located on the extracellular surface of the cell membrane,
while Dayton and Schollmeyer (5) reported its presence at the
cytoplasmic surface of the cell membrane of cultured myoblast.
In a cross-section of the cryostat specimen, most of the
soluble CANP was removed during washing. A small portion,
however, seemed to be attached to the cell membrane in both
normal and dystrophic chicken. We find it difficult to conclude whether the fluorescence at the cell membrane is inside
or outside of the surface membrane.

We have already demonstrated the presence of CANP at the
Z-band of the chicken myofibrils (6) as confirmed by Dayton
and his group (5). In human glycerinated myofibrils, CANP is
also localized at the Z-band. The CANP bound to the Z-band
was extracted from washed chicken myofibrils by a buffer of
low ionic strength and accounted for approximately 4% of that
contained in the whole muscle homogenate (6). The myofibril-
bound CANP was partially purified as previously described (6).
The concentration of Ca ion for half-maximum activation was
0.18 mM. This value indicates that the myofibril-bound enzyme
is more sensitive to Ca ion than the soluble one (7).
Ouchterlony's immunodiffusion method disclosed a cross reaction between soluble and myofibril-bound CANP (6). When primary cultured cells of fibroblast were used, diffuse fluorescence was observed throughout the cytoplasm, but faint fluorescence was also observed apparently associated with the
filamentous structure (8). In peripheral nerve, the axons
were homogenously stained with antibody against CANP. An

electron microscopic study to determine whether CANP is bound
with neurofilament or other cytoskeleton is now under way.

The association of CANP with cytoskeleton in the central
nervous system is less clear.   Ca-activated protease was
reported by Ishizaki and his group (9) to be specific to the
160K-dalton component of the neurofilament triplet and is
associated with the neurofilament enriched cytoskeleton of the
spinal cord in physiological ionic strength; it is dissociated
in the presence of 0.6 M KCl.   In our immunoblotting study,
the presence of CANP was not confirmed in extracted neurofilament, but this does not necessarily mean that CANP is not
bound to the neurofilament (10).

Recently Sato and Miyatake (11) reported that incubation
of purified myelin extracted from human brain in 1 mM $CaCl_2$
resulted in the degradation of basic protein.   The E-64-a
partially inhibited its degradation.   They found that incubation of myelin itself without addition of Ca ion also resulted
in the digestion of basic protein (12).   The intrinsic concentration of Ca ion in the myelin itself is 25 μM.   This
finding suggests that purified human myelin contains both m
and μ types of CANP-like enzymes which mainly degrade basic
protein.   These results give strong support to the premise of
the association of CANP with cytoskeleton in the central nervous system, but there is so far no direct evidence of its
presence.

III. EFFECT OF CANP ON PURIFIED CYTOSKELETON

In 1975 Dayton's group reported that CANP had no effect on
myosin, actin and α-actinin, but that it easily digested
C-protein, tropomyosin and troponin (13).   Table I shows a
summary of the effect of CANP on various cytoskeletons (7,
13-20).

We have studied the effect of both m- and μ-CANP extracted
from bovine liver on cytoskeleton.   The specific activity of
both was adjusted by caseinolytic activity.   Among muscle proteins, troponin T (TN-T) and C-protein were most sensitive,
desmin and TN-I were moderately digested, but actin, TN-C and
α-actinin were resistant.   In brain proteins, microtubule-
associated proteins (MAPs) were most sensitive and tubulin was
less sensitive.   The m- and μ-CANP are qualitatively similar
in digesting the cytoskeleton, but, m-CANP seemed to be more
potent to cytoskeleton than μ-CANP as shown in Table II.

The effect of CANP extracted from peripheral nerve on the
neurofilament triplet extracted from the same peripheral nerve
was then studied.   Incubation of crude m-CANP extracted from
the sciatic nerve with neurofilament triplet revealed almost

TABLE I. Digestion of Various Cytoskeletons by m-CANP

	M.W.	Mode of Digestion	Authors (reference)	
Myosin H chain	200,000	partly degraded	Sugita et al.	1980 (17)
L chain 1	24,000	partly degraded to 22,000	Ishiura et al.	1982 (7)
2	20,000	no effect	Sugita et al.	1980 (17)
3	16,000	no effect	Sugita et al.	1980 (17)
Actin	42,000	no effect	Dayton et al.	1975 (13)
Tropomyosin	33,000	degraded to 13,000 – 18,000	Dayton et al.	1975 (13)
Troponin T	42,000	degraded	Ishiura et al.	1979 (18)
I	20,000	degraded	Ishiura et al.	1979 (18)
C	17,000	no effect	Dayton et al.	1975 (13)
M-protein	165,000	no effect	Ishiura et al.	1982 (7)
C-protein	135,000	degraded	Dayton et al.	1975 (13)
α-Actinin	96,000	partly degraded to 78,000	Ishiura et al.	1982 (7)
Filamin	250,000	degraded to 240,000	Davies et al.	1978 (14)

Protein		Effect	Reference		
Band 3	600,000	degraded	Maruyama	1981	(19)
Connectin	1,000,000	no effect	Maruyama	1981	(19)
Desmin	55,000	degraded	Ishiura et al.	1982	(7)
Vimentin	58,000	degraded	Nelson & Traub	1981	(15)
Z-protein	54,000	no effect	Ishiura et al.	1982	(7)
Myelin basic protein	19,000	degraded	Yanagisawa et al.	1983	(20)
Wolfgram protein	54,000 62,000	no effect	Yanagisawa et al.	1983	(20)
Proteolipid protein	25,000	no effect	Yanagisawa et al.	1983	(20)
MAPs	340,000 300,000	degraded	Malik et al.	1981	(16)
Neurofilament	200,000 160,000 68,000	degraded	Malik et al.	1981	(16)
Tubulin	52,000	degraded	Ishiura et al.	1979	(18)

TABLE II.   Effect of m- and μ-CANP on Cytoskeleton

	m-CANP	μ-CANP
Muscle protein		
Myosin H chain	+	$\pm$
L chain 1	+	$\pm$
2	−	−
3	−	−
Actin	−	−
Tropomyosin	++	++
Troponin T	+++	++
I	++	+
C	−	−
α-Actinin	−	−
C-protein	++	+
Desmin	++	+
Brain protein		
MAPs	+++	+++
Neurofilament 200K	+	+
Protein 160K	+++	++
68K	++	+
Tubulin	++	++

+, digested;   −, no effect

simultaneous disappearance of triplet subunits and inhibition
by E-64-c (10,21). We have also demonstrated the presence of
μ-CANP activity in the peripheral nerve, which preferentially
degraded the 160K component. The triplet was degraded in the
order of 160K, 68K and 200K components, respectively (22).
E-64-c suppressed the degradation of the neurofilament.

IV. INCUBATION EXPERIMENT

In order to study the role of m- and μ-CANP in living vertebrate tissues, an attempt was made to control the cytosolic
calcium concentration by ionophore A23187 in vitro. As
already reported (7), rat soleus incubated in 1 mM Ca ion with

25 μg/ml of A23187 for 3 hr electronmicroscopically revealed the preferential disappearance of the Z-band but relative preservation of the M-line. Sodium dodecyl sulfate (SDS) gel electrophoresis revealed a marked decrease in α-actinin in calcium-treated muscle and an increase in the substance released into the medium. Addition of E-64-c partly suppressed the release of α-actinin (7). To clarify whether μ-CANP is active in the physiological condition, a similar experiment was performed using 10^{-3} or 10^{-4} M Ca ion with 2 μM of A23187 as was used in the experiment by Rodemann et al. (23) for 3 hr.

As shown in Table III, the amount of released tyrosine increased in the medium with Ca ion, more prominently in 10^{-3} M than 10^{-4} M. Additionally, tyrosine release was partly inhibited by addition of E-64-c (25 μM) but not indomethacin (2.8 μM) (Table IV). If intracellular Ca ion concentration after 3 hr incubation is about equal to extracellular concentration, this result is not incompatible with the idea that the μ-CANP in soleus plays the same role in the muscle protein degradation. Further experimentation is necessary before a final conclusion is reached.

A similar experiment was carried out using a short segment of rat sciatic nerve. Fresh rat sciatic nerve was transected and divided into 6 mm segments and each segment was incubated in various amounts of Ca ion and 1% of Triton X-100 in vitro. A selective loss of neurofilament triplet was observed in medium containing mM order of Ca ion and inhibited in the presence of E-64-c (24). When the segment of sciatic nerve was incubated for 5 hr in the presence of 50 μM or 0.1 mM of

TABLE III. Effect of Ca Ion Concentration in the Medium on the Increase in Protein Degradation

Ca^{2+} concentration	Protein degradation n mol Tyr/mg/3 hr	% increase
Control	0.388 ± 0.010	
10^{-4}M	0.424 ± 0.012* (n = 23)	10
10^{-3}M	0.591 ± 0.019** (n = 24)	52

(Mean $\pm$ S.D), *: $p < 0.05$, **: $p < 0.001$

TABLE IV.   Effect of E-64-c and Indomethacin on the Increase
in Protein Degradation

Ca^{2+} concentration	Protein degradation	% inhibition
Ca free	0.388 ± 0.010 (n = 28)	
+E-64-c	0.339 ± 0.012 (n = 12)	15
10^{-4} M Ca	0.424 ± 0.012 (n = 23)	
+E-64-c	0.361 ± 0.010 (n = 16)	15
+Indomethacin	0.420 ± 0.013 (n = 8)	0
10^{-3} M Ca	0.591 ± 0.019 (n = 24)	
+E-64-c	0.495 ± 0.046 (n = 8)	16
+Indomethacin	0.560 ± 0.037 (n = 8)	5

Ca ion, the degradation of each component of neurofilament was
not clear. The main reason for the negative result might be
the lower content of CANP in peripheral nerve compared with
skeletal muscle (19) (1/30) and lower specific activity of
μ-CANP compared to m-CANP.

V. ROLE OF CANP IN MUSCLE PROTEIN DEGRADATION IN PATHOLOGICAL STATES

In 1976 Kar and Pearson (25) reported an increase in Ca-
activated neutral protease activities in Duchenne muscular
dystrophy (DMD) muscle, suggesting the role of this enzyme in

muscle protein degradation. Since then, several workers have reported an increase in CANP activity in various muscle diseases, but not in denervation atrophy as shown in Table V (25-31). When we look at the DMD muscle, different stages of the degradation were visible, from apparently normal muscle fiber and opaque fiber, which was supposed to be an early stage of degeneration with hypercontraction of myofibril and increased Ca ion concentration by the histochemical method, to disappearance of muscle fiber due to the invasion of macrophages.

Questions then arise as to what stage and kind of role CANP plays in successive processes of muscle protein degradation. To clarify this, we induced acute muscle degeneration in rat soleus by direct intramuscular injection of myotoxic substances, one plasmocid (32,33) and the other a local anesthetic (bupivacaine or Marcaine) as the model of muscle necrosis (34-36). One of the main lesion sites is supposed to be the surface membrane. These toxins can produce the homogenous degeneration of the entire soleus muscle.

Two hr after treatment with 1 mg Marcaine, the density of the Z-band was markedly decreased (35). In accordance with this finding, preferential decrease in α-actinin was observed. At 24 hr, other structural proteins began to sharply decrease simultaneously. Almost all the structural proteins had disappeared and were degraded into smaller molecular weight products at 48 hr. A 43K dalton protein identified as actin, however, was resistant to degradation. The decrease in α-actinin at 3 hr after injection was suppressed by the coinjection of a protease inhibitor, E-64-c, suggesting that cysteine-dependent protease removed α-actinin from the Z-band.

Two hr after injection of 2 mg of plasmocid, α-actinin content had already decreased to 1/4 that of control, and had almost disappeared 12 hr after injection. Other proteins, tropomyosin and heavy chain of myosin were also gradually decreased in amount. The decrease in α-actinin was partially suppressed by coinjection of EGTA or E-64-c with plasmocid (33,34).

Examination of the time course of the lysosomal enzymes, cathepsin B and L in Marcaine injected muscle followed. The specific activity was almost the same as that of control 6 hr after the injection, when the preferential decrease in α-actinin had already occurred. The same was true in the case of plasmocid. The activity of cathepsin B and L, however, began to increase and reached the peak level which was 13 times higher than the control after 48 hr (Table VI). The change of activity seemed proportional to the number of invading cells detected by the histochemical technique. These results suggested a close relationship between the increase in cathepsin B and L and the decrease in structural proteins in

TABLE V. Ca-activated Neutral Protease in Pathological States

Authors (reference)	Material & Method	Disease	Result (%)
Kar & Pearson 1976 (25)	muscle homogenate	DMD Denervating diseases	270 no change
Ebashi & Sugita 1979 (26)	partial purification	DMD Neurogenic atrophy	150 no change
Dayton et al. 1979 (27)	P_0–40 fraction	Vit. E deficiency	360
Neerunjun & Dubowitz 1979 (28)	supernatant particulate fraction	Dystrophic hamster Dystrophic mouse	150–200 200–300
Sugita et al. 1982 (29)	partial purification	Dystrophic chicken	160–180
Elce et al. 1983 (30)	supernatant (solid phase immunoassay)	Denervation	140–180
Kimura et al. 1983 (31)	supernatant (ELISA)	Dystrophic chicken	150

TABLE VI. Effect of Coadministration of Cycloheximide (CHI)
and Bupivacaine on Lysosomal Enzyme Activities
and Amount of Structural Proteins in Soleus Muscle
48 hr after Bupivacaine Administration.

Enzymes	Specific Activity (Units/mg)		
	Bupivacaine (B)	Control (C)	B + CHI
Cathepsins B & L	314±16*	24±3	72±14*
Cathepsin D	0.499±0.042*	0.163±0.013	0.205±0.018*
α-glucosidase	1.85±0.19	2.20±0.12	0.64±0.05*
α-galactosidase	3.89±0.36*	1.03±0.08	1.37±0.10*
Acid phosphatase	0.175±0.011	0.174±0.008	0.122±0.009*
Non-collagen protein (mg/soleus)	4.03±0.29*	9.08±0.74	6.87±0.26*

From ref. 35. Results are presented as mean ± SEM (n=10).
*p<0.01 (B vs. C ; B + CHI vs. B)

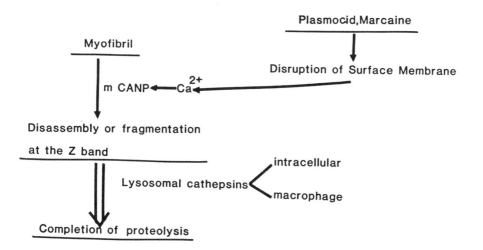

FIGURE 1. Proposed mechanism of muscle protein degradation in plasmocid or Marcaine induced muscle necrosis.

treated muscle. The localization of cathepsin B in Marcaine treated muscle was investigated using an immunofluorescence technique. The fluorescence labeled antibody against this enzyme was demonstrated in the macrophages (34), but the intramuscular nerve and degenerating muscle fibers were almost unstainable. At this stage of necrosis, i.e., 48 hr after Marcaine injection, most of the infiltrated cells were identified as macrophages by electron microscopy (34). Basophilic mast cells were rarely found histochemically.

If the cathepsins derived from the macrophages play a major role in protein degradation in a later stage, the enzyme activities in Marcaine-injected, cycloheximide-treated muscle should be lower than those of Marcaine-injected one. As shown in Table VI, intraperitoneal injection of 1 ml of 2 mM cyclo-heximide simultaneous with Marcaine administration signifi-cantly depressed the drastic increase in various enzymes induced by Marcaine (36). The decrease in the content of structural proteins 48 hr after Marcaine treatment was suppressed to 56% after cycloheximide administration (Table VI) (36). Concomitant with this finding, cycloheximide admin-istered muscles were shown not to be infiltrated by macro-phages.

Based on the results thus obtained, the mechanism of muscle protein degradation is illustrated in Fig. 1. In both plasmocid and Marcaine injection, intracellular concentration of Ca ion has been found high enough to activate m-CANP by histochemical method due to disruption of the surface membrane by myotoxic substances. It should be specifically mentioned that no lysosomal enzymes tested were increased at the initial stage of muscle degeneration, i.e., 3 hr after injection. Thus, we concluded that Ca-activated protease digested and removed the Z-band at the early stage of muscle protein degra-dation prior to massive degradation of myofilaments.

At the later stage of muscle degradation, the dramatic increase in the activity of lysosomal cathepsins was intimate-ly correlated with the disappearance of overall muscle pro-tein. Despite the lack of direct evidence, it seems reason-able to conclude that the muscle protein degradation is caused mainly by the enhancement of cathepsin activity. Surprisingly, the localization of one of the cathepsins, cathepsin B, was limited to invading phagocytes. The number of phagocytes increased in proportion to the cathepsin ac-tivity, suggesting that the activity of cathepsin B and L in the muscle homogenate at the later stage of muscle degenera-tion is perhaps derived from invaded cells. The cycloheximide experiment confirmed this.

In many pathological states, e.g. human muscular dystrophy and ischemia, decrease or disappearance of the Z-band is a common phenomenon which may be caused by CANP activated by a massive influx of extracellular Ca ion due to disrupted surface membrane.

This causes fragmentation or disassembly of the myofibril so that it becomes accessible to further proteolysis. The later stage of protein degradation is accomplished by lysosomal cathepsins, probably derived from invaded macrophage which was triggered by the fragmentation of myofibril by CANP.

REFERENCES

1. Suzuki, K., Tsuji, S., Kubota, S., Kimura, Y., and Imahori, K., J. Biochem. 90:275 (1981).
2. Tsujinaka, T., Sakon, M., Kambayashi, J., and Kosaki, G., Thrombosis Res. 28:149 (1982).
3. Murachi, T., Tanaka, K., Hatanaka, M., and Murakami, T., in "Advances in Enzyme Regulation" (G. Weber, ed.), p. 407. Pergamon Press, New York, 1981.
4. Barth, R., and Elce, J. S., Am. J. Physiol. 240:E493 (1981).
5. Dayton, W. R., and Schollmeyer, J. V., Exp. Cell Res. 136:423 (1981).
6. Ishiura, S., Sugita, H., Nonaka, I., and Imahori, K., J. Biochem. 87:343 (1980).
7. Ishiura, S., Nonaka, I., and Sugita, H., in "Muscular Dystrophy" (S. Ebashi, ed.), p. 265. University of Tokyo Press, Tokyo, 1982.
8. Ishiura, S., unpublished result.
9. Ishizaki, Y., Tashiro, T., and Kurokawa, M., Eur. J. Biochem. 131:41 (1983).
10. Kamakura, K., Ishiura, S., Sugita, H., and Toyokura, Y., Biomed. Res. 3:91 (1982).
11. Sato, S., and Miyatake, T., Biomed. Res. 3:461 (1982).
12. Sato, S., Yanagisawa, K., and Miyatake, T., Neurochem. Res. 9:629 (1984).
13. Dayton, W. R., Goll, D. E., Stromer, M. H., Reville, W. J., Zeece, M. G., and Robson, R. M., in "Protease and Biological Control" (E. Reich, et al., eds.), p. 551. Cold Spring Harbor Laboratory, New York, 1975.
14. Davies, P. J. A., Wallach, D., Willingham, M. C., and Pastan, I., J. Biol. Chem. 253:4036 (1978).
15. Nelson, W. J., and Traub, P., Eur. J. Biochem. 116:51 (1981).
16. Malik, M. N., Meyers, L. A., Iqbal, K., Sheikh, A. M., Scotto, L., and Wisniewski, H. M., Life Sci. 29:792 (1981).
17. Sugita, H., Ishiura, S., Suzuki, K., and Imahori, K., Muscle and Nerve 3:335 (1980).

18. Ishiura, S., Sugita, H., Suzuki, K., and Imahori, K., J. Biochem. 86:579 (1979).
19. Maruyama, K., J. Biochem. 89:711 (1981).
20. Yanagisawa, K., Sato, S., Amaya, N., and Miyatake, T., Neurochem. Res. 8:1285 (1983).
21. Kamakura, K., Ishiura, S., Sugita, H., and Toyokura, Y., J. Neurochem. 40:908 (1983).
22. Kamakura, K., unpublished result.
23. Rodemann, H. P., Waxman, L., and Goldberg, A. L., J. Biol. Chem. 257:8716 (1982).
24. Kamakura, K., Ihara, Y., Sugita, H., and Toyokura, Y., Biomed. Res. 2:327 (1981).
25. Kar, N. C., and Pearson, C. M., Clin. Chim. Acta. 73:293 (1976).
26. Ebashi, S., and Sugita, H., in "Current Topics in Nerve and Muscle Research" (A. J. Aguayo, et al., eds.), p. 73. Excerpta Medica, Amsterdam - Oxford, 1979.
27. Dayton, W. R., Schollmeyer, J. V., Chan, A. C., and Allen, C. E., Biochim. Biophys. Acta 584:216 (1979).
28. Neerunjun, J. S., and Dubowitz, V., J. Neurol. Sci. 40:105 (1979).
29. Sugita, H., Kimura, M., Tarumoto, Y., Tamai, M., Hanada, K., Ishiura, S., Nonaka, I., Ohzeki, M., and Imahori, K., Muscle and Nerve 5:738 (1982).
30. Elce, J. S., Hasspieler, R., and Boegman, R. J., Exp. Neurol. 81:320 (1983).
31. Kimura, K., Imajyo, S., Suzuki, K., and Imahori, K., Seikagaku (in Japanese) 55:977 (1983).
32. Nakase, H., unpublished result.
33. Ishiura, S., and Sugita, H., in "Molecular Aspect of Neurological Disorders" (L. Austin, ed.), p. 29. Academic Press, Australia, 1983.
34. Ishiura, S., Nonaka, I., Nakase, H., Tsuchiya, K., Okada, S., and Sugita, H., J. Biochem. 94:311 (1983).
35. Nonaka, I., Takagi, A., Ishiura, S., Nakase, H., and Sugita, H., Acta Neuropath. 60:167 (1983).
36. Ishiura, S., Nonaka, I., Fujita, T., and Sugita, H., J. Biochem. 94:1631 (1983).

INDEX